Everything
Elderberry

Everything
Elderberry

How to Forage, Cultivate, and Cook with this Amazing Natural Remedy

Susannah Shmurak

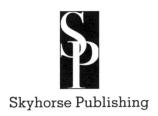

Skyhorse Publishing

Skyhorse Publishing books may be purchased in bulk at special discounts for sales promotion, corporate gifts, fund-raising, or educational purposes. Special editions can also be created to specifications. For details, contact the Special Sales Department, Skyhorse Publishing, 307 West 36th Street, 11th Floor, New York, NY 10018 or info@skyhorsepublishing.com.

Skyhorse® and Skyhorse Publishing® are registered trademarks of Skyhorse Publishing, Inc.®, a Delaware corporation.

Visit our website at www.skyhorsepublishing.com.

10 9 8 7 6 5 4

Library of Congress Cataloging-in-Publication Data is available on file.

Cover design by Daniel Brount
Cover photos by Susannah Shmurak and Jan Berry

Print ISBN: 978-1-5107-5400-3
Ebook ISBN: 978-1-5107-5401-0

Printed in China

TABLE OF CONTENTS

ELDERFLOWER AND ELDERBERRY RECIPES 97

PART I: PREPARATIONS FOR IMMUNE SUPPORT 97

PART II: ELDERBERRY AND ELDERFLOWER DESSERTS, TREATS & MORE 117

INTRODUCTION

While modern medicine has in many cases eclipsed tried-and-true herbal remedies, another modern invention, the internet, has helped revive these fading ways to treat illness and support everyday good health. You probably picked up this book because you read about elderberry syrup on a blog and were curious to know more. That's how I first learned about elderberries, too.

Reading about elderberry syrup online immediately piqued my interest. A simple berry-based concoction that could help me fight off colds and flu was *very* appealing in a region of the country where winter (and cold season!) lasts five to six long months.

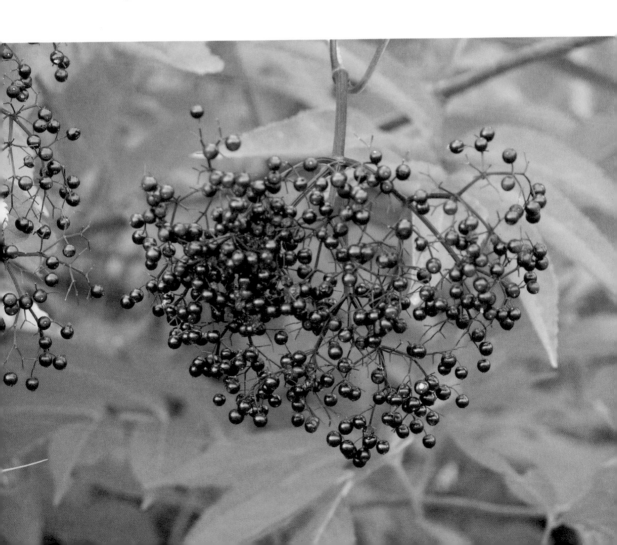

But buying tiny, expensive bottles of elderberry syrup did not appeal to this frugal do-it-yourselfer, and I quickly schooled myself in ways to tap the benefits of elderberries without breaking the bank. As I learned to make my own elderberry preparations, I developed an insatiable curiosity about other herbal remedies. Exploring the fascinating world of plant medicine, I discovered hundreds of common plants—some masquerading as weeds in our gardens, some staples of the spice cabinet—that we can use to address common ailments. Many of these simple herbs and spices show up in the recipes included here.

This book also contains information on how to source elderberries and use them safely, as well as what scientific evidence we have for their storied health benefits. In my effort to understand this intriguing plant better, I sought out scientists, growers, herbalists, and makers of jams and spirits. I combed through historical herbal texts, centuries' worth of cookbooks, and piles of modern herbalist books. I experimented with using the flowers and berries in baking, teas, and condiments, and plied family and friends with the results. It's all here for you, along with loads of information about how to find or grow elderflowers and elderberries and how you can use these ages-old remedies in your wellness routine.

Elderberry has served for many as a gateway to the not-quite lost—and, thanks to the internet and ever-growing popular interest, quickly rebounding—art of home remedies. Since elderberry has been widely studied, is readily available, and tastes so good, it's a perfect place to start if you're curious about supporting health naturally.

How to Use This Book

Whether you're a veteran forager, an enthusiastic gardener, or someone who just wants to understand what all the fuss is about, this book has you covered.

You can absolutely use this book just for the how-to's on health-supporting teas, tinctures, and other herbal concoctions, or peruse the recipes to discover how versatile elderberry can be. For those readers interested in learning more about elder's rich history, foraging and growing information, or the scientific studies conducted on elderberry, I've provided overviews. Since there are so many conflicting recommendations about how to use elderberry, I spent a lot of time sifting through herbal reference books and speaking with herbalists and biochemists. You'll find what I gleaned in the section on using elderberry for immune support.

>> **Please do not skip the section on safely preparing and using elderberries and elderflowers, and if you plan to forage, the section on correctly identifying elderberry plants.** Though elderberry is a food, there are some important things to know in order to use it safely and effectively.

While elderberry syrup is perhaps this impressive little berry's best-known form, there is so much more we can make from flavorful elderberries! In addition to their uses for immune support, elderberries contain potent antioxidants that support long-term health, and they make nutritious and tasty additions to baked goods, drinks, and all manner of treats. Once you get started making your own elderberry gummies and homemade beverages, you'll likely find lots more ways to incorporate this delicious ingredient into everyday cooking.

As you'll discover in the pages that follow, elderflowers also have a long history of medicinal and culinary use. If you've never cooked with flowers before, get ready to have some fun with elder's beautiful and delicious blossoms.

Dive into some of the history and research, check out the foraging and growing information, or just whip up some syrup, muffins, tea, or jam from these gorgeous and tasty fruits and flowers. Enjoy!

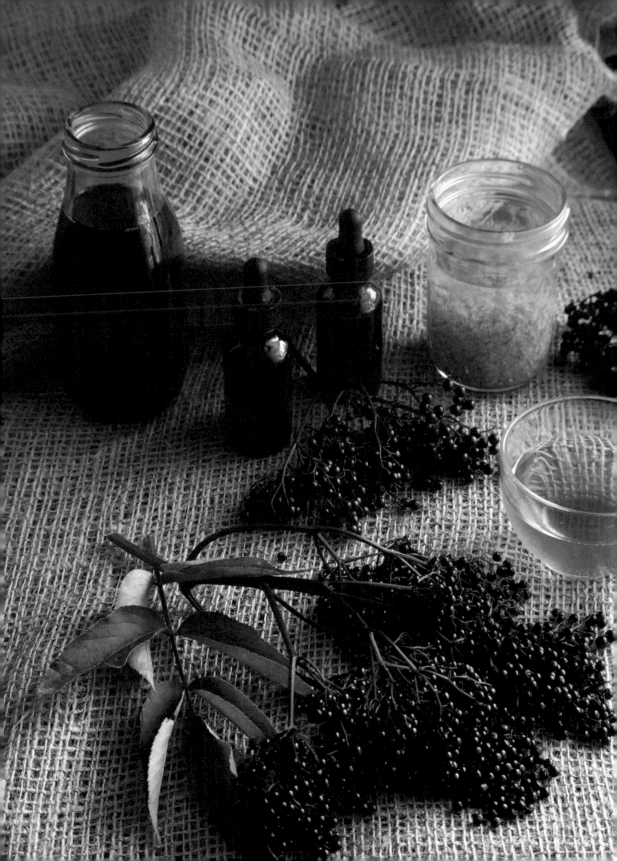

CHAPTER 1

AN ELDERBERRY PRIMER

"SAMBUCUS CANADENSIS. *ELDER* . . . In domestic medicine, this plant
forms almost a pharmacy in itself."
—Charles Millspaugh, *American Medicinal Plants* (1892)[1]

Let's start at the beginning. What is elderberry, anyway?

Elderberry is the common name for the fruit of the plant *Sambucus*, varieties
of which grow in many parts of the world, from Australia to Canada. Common
names include elder, black elderberry, European elderberry, blue elderberry,
elder bush, and hundreds of others in dozens of languages. The French call it
sureau noir, the Danish call it *hyld*, and the Germans call it *schwarzer Holunder*.
In Italian it's *sambuco*, in Spanish *saúco*, in Swedish *fläder*, in Farsi *palam*, and
in Russian *busine*. In various times and places it has also been known as Judas
tree, bore tree, pipe tree, and Devil's wood, among many others.

It's the European variety, *Sambucus nigra*, you're most likely to have sampled as dry berries or in bottled syrup. Not many people realize that North
America has its very own subspecies of elderberry called *Sambucus canadensis*,
which grows in the northeastern part of the continent, and *Sambucus cerulea*,
which grows in the west. In desert locations, *Sambucus cerulea* often goes by
the name *mexicana*. Other parts of the world have additional subspecies. In
South America, the native *Sambucus australis* is used in much the same way as
Europeans have used *nigra* for centuries. Numerous additional kinds of elderberry grow in Asia and the Middle East.

The common name English speakers use derives from the Anglo-Saxon *aeld*,
meaning fire, though exactly why isn't certain. A number of sources suggest
that the hollow stems of the elder were used as blowing tubes to kindle fire or
perhaps for smoking, while herbalist Matthew Wood speculates the name may
have had to do with elder's common use as a fever-reducer.[2] The wood of elder,
which has an easy-to-remove-pith, was also used both by Native Americans

---

1   Charles Millspaugh, *American Medicinal Plants* (New York: Boericke & Tafel, 1892), 75–6.
2   Matthew Wood, *The Book of Herbal Wisdom: Using Plants as Medicine.* (Berkeley: North Atlantic
     Books, 1997), 425.

and Europeans for making children's toys such as popguns, as well as musical instruments. The Greek root *sambuke* and Latin *sambucus* refer to ancient musical instruments made from elder wood.

Elder shrubs and trees produce copious blooms of beautiful and deliciously-scented flowers in early summer and gorgeous rich clusters of drooping elderberries in late summer to fall. The fresh berries from many plants you'll find don't taste like much on their own, but cooked down and sweetened they make a rich flavoring that's been used in everything from jams and pies to sauces and wines. You'll find recipes for all of these in the second half of this book.

Most of what we know about elderberries comes from studies on the variety grown in Europe, where elderberry has a long tradition of use as "the country people's medicine chest." Herbal books dating back centuries inform us that elderberry and elderflower, as well as elder bark and leaves, have been used as folk medicine for a wide variety of ailments. Elder's popularity in Europe never waned, and if you stop in at many European pharmacies, you'll likely find numerous elderberry and elderflower cold remedies, from tonics to throat lozenges. You may have had some without even realizing it: the popular Swiss brand Ricola includes elderflowers in many of its cough drops, available at many American drug stores.

In North America, Native Americans also used elder to treat a wide array of illnesses. Recent research into the North American varieties suggests that they possess similar medicinal properties to their European cousins, and the dozens of ways North American tribes employed elder closely resemble those used in ancient Greece and Renaissance Europe. Comparable uses have also been documented in Latin American folk medicine and traditional Chinese medicine.

As interest in the healing power of foods has grown, elderberries have gotten special attention for their exceptionally high concentration of anthocyanins, the compounds in dark fruits like blueberries and black currants that give them their deep purple color. Anthocyanins have shown promise in lab studies for protecting our bodies from what's known as oxidative stress, which is linked with diseases like cancer and brain degeneration as well as accelerated aging. Research continues to yield information about other potentially beneficial compounds found in the berries and flowers.

Elderberry's current claim to fame, though, stems from the publicity it got when human trials in the 1990s suggested that elderberry extract could significantly shorten the duration and severity of flu, further supported in the years since by human, animal, and *in vitro* studies. Since then, supplement makers have launched scores of elderberry-based products meant to be taken medicinally, as they have been for centuries by home-remedy makers in Europe, the Americas, and other parts of the world. According to the National Center for Complementary and Integrative Health, sales of elderberry supplements rose by 50 percent between 2003 and 2008. Market reports from the American Botanical Council show growth in sales of 138 percent in 2018.[3]

An online search will yield hundreds of options for syrups, extracts, gummies, juices, tinctures, and herbal blends meant to treat or prevent respiratory illness. The price tag on a small jar of gummies (sometimes $25!) speaks to the market that has sprung up for the "immune-boosting" abilities of these tasty little berries. Learning to prepare your own elderberry concoctions will save you quite a bit over buying these pricey products, and if you learn to forage or grow your own, you may enjoy the benefit of this delicious medicinal berry for free.

Elderberries have become so popular that the last few years have seen shortages, with growers unable to meet the demand. Currently, more than 95 percent of commercial elderberries come from Europe, but enthusiastic North American growers have seen an excellent opportunity and hope to make greater contributions to the world supply of elderberries.

Though currently less prominent than the berry in many parts of the world, the flower historically has been has been viewed as more medicinally powerful, used commonly as a treatment for fever and a variety of other ailments. Finding elderflowers in early summer and drying them for winter use is easy, fun, and will save money. They impart a lovely flavor to all kinds of drinks, from teas to cocktails, and elderflower syrup can be used to make delicious frozen treats and cakes. Research has shown elder blossoms to be rich in antioxidants, and elderflower tea has long been herbalists' go-to remedy for fevers and colds.

Elderflower's abilities to soften and heal skin makes it a popular addition to skin salves, especially useful for older skin (see recipes beginning on page 173). According to herbalist Matthew Wood, a cooled infusion of elderflowers can also be used as an eye rinse, or applied as a compress for sprains, bruises, and sore muscles.[4]

---

3 "NIH Announces Five Botanical Research Centers," National Center for Complementary and Integrative Health, Aug 31, 2010. nccih.nih.gov/news/2010/083110.htm and 2018 Market Report, American Botanical Council cms.herbalgram.org/herbalgram/issue123/files/HG123-HMR.pdf
4 Wood, *Herbal Wisdom*, 433.

Even the leaves, which may make you very ill if consumed, are useful topically and have a long history of medicinal applications, as you'll see in the section on the plant's historical uses.

One of the most appealing things about elderberries is that unlike many so-called superfoods, they grow wild in much of the world, so they're easy to source inexpensively. No need to spend exorbitant amounts of money to have a potent home remedy at the ready. Better still, the concoctions you can make with elderflower and elderberry taste *amazing*!

So whether you're a long-time user of elderberry syrup or you've never even noticed the stuff on your grocery store's shelves, elderberry is a fantastic tool to add to (or launch) your home herbal arsenal. Read on to find out why.

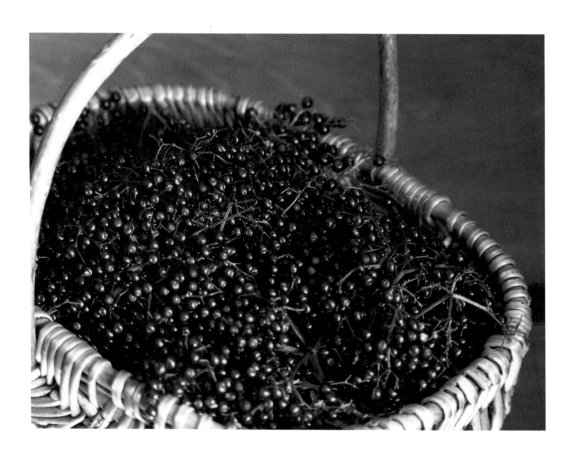

The Usefulness of Herbal Medicine in the Modern World

While modern medicine and folk remedies seem to be at opposite ends of a spectrum, in fact many modern drugs derive from plants that researchers explored precisely because of their long history as folk medicine. A large percentage of modern pharmaceuticals were developed from plant-based medicines, and scientists continue to identify medicinally-useful plants that may help fight disease and support health.

Though not every herbal preparation has been thoroughly studied using modern scientific methods, more studies come out each year that shed light on why people have turned to these plants for centuries. Type the name of an herb into the National Institutes of Health PubMed database, and you'll find there's a great deal of interest in better understanding how these traditional remedies work, from commonplace cinnamon and mint to less familiar herbs that have gained popularity for treating a range of conditions, like St. John's Wort and gingko.

While verifying a plant's biological activity with science is certainly valuable, we shouldn't dismiss folk remedies just because they don't yet have the scientific studies proving their effectiveness. With thousands of plants used medicinally around the world, it's simply not possible to have incontrovertible scientific proof of how or if they all work. Given the rising interest in plant-based medicine, odds are someone's working on a study as you read these words. Herbalists have passed down centuries of plant wisdom, and some excellent recent books aim to make that wisdom accessible to an ever-growing number of us looking to support health with plants.

Just to be clear: I am *not* suggesting you reject conventional medicine altogether! It certainly has its place, especially in acute situations. But as evidence mounts that the foods we eat and our lifestyle choices greatly affect our health, the conventional medical community has begun to embrace elements of natural health as well. More doctors are prescribing time outdoors, for instance, as our intuitive sense that contact with nature is good for our well-being is borne out by scientific research. The American Academy of Pediatrics now recommends an old folk remedy for coughs—honey—and advises against giving children over-the-counter cough medicines.

Though the dominance of modern science has made many skeptical of herbal remedies, you've probably at some point in your life found relief thanks to herbal wisdom passed down from time immemorial. That cup of chamomile tea to help you unwind or the ginger you take for nausea are both longstanding herbal remedies.

A glance at the herbal tea aisle in any grocery store demonstrates how mainstream many of these ideas have become in the last few decades. Whether it's a sleepytime tea or some of the many options from Traditional Medicinals (founded by renowned herbalist Rosemary Gladstar, sometimes referred to as the "godmother of modern herbalism"), addressing some common ailments from the sniffles to insomnia with simple herbs we sip from a cup is within reach for all of us.

Simple kitchen ingredients have been used to help prevent and treat illness for centuries. Along with honey, cinnamon can soothe coughs, while thyme's antimicrobial abilities make thyme-derived botanical disinfectants as effective as bleach.[5] Our great-grandmothers knew many of these once-common uses for everyday plants, and a new generation of herbalists is working to re-familiarize us with this age-old knowledge.

Consider adding the power of elderberry to your arsenal of gentle herbs that can help support better health. Whether or not you're ready to dive into the fascinating world of herbal remedies, you don't have much to lose with these tasty berries and flowers, which also have a long history of culinary use because they're delicious as well as medicinal.

While you need to understand how to source and use your elderberries safely, you don't need to be a trained herbalist to try some of these simple elderberry-based home remedies. When you start exploring the power of plants, you'll likely find yourself drawn to the ways you can use common kitchen ingredients—like ginger or cloves, for example—to support wellness. You'll find a number of these oft-overlooked but potent spices included in some of the elderberry recipes to increase their health-promoting properties. I've also included a list of useful books and websites on herbal subjects in the resources section if you'd like to learn about other medicinal plants.

The next section looks at elderberry's intriguing history as a multi-purpose herbal medicine. The following chapter examines what modern science can tell us about how elderberry works, in many cases bearing out these historical uses.

---

5 "EPA Registered Hard Surface Disinfectants Comparison Chart" education.nh.gov/instruction /school_health/documents/disinfectants.pdf

A Brief(ish) Look at Elderberry's Long History of Medicinal Use

While elderberry is new to many of us, it's been a go-to remedy for a wide range of ailments for millenia, and as you'll discover, modern scientific research has supported many of these historical applications. Common folk and physicians have used various parts of the elder medicinally for more than two thousand years. Large numbers of elderberry seeds have been found at archaeological excavations dating back thousands of years, suggesting that elder already had a place in the regular diets, and possibly apothecaries, of prehistoric peoples.[6]

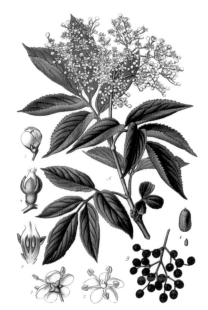

Amédée Masclef, 1891, from *Atlas des plantes de France*

The references to medicinal uses of elder in historical texts are so numerous, I've included only a small selection to give you a sense of this remarkable plant's varied use over the centuries as a "people's medicine chest," a pharmacy for treating an impressive array of complaints. Several Greek and Roman medical sources mention the elder's bark, leaves, flowers, and berries as effective remedies for maladies as diverse as dyspepsia and snake bite. Ancient Greeks used elder for a range of health issues, and the "father of medicine," Hippocrates (c. 460–370 BC) suggested the leaves and berries for numerous medical problems, reportedly declaring elder a "medicine chest in itself" and a "plant from the gods."

Greek physician and botanist Dioscorides (c. 40–90 AD) explored the medical uses of hundreds of plants in his five-volume *De Materia Medica* (*On Medical Material*), a precursor to modern pharmacopeias that circulated continuously in hand-copied manuscripts for fifteen centuries. The entry on *chamaiacte*, translated as dwarf elder (*Sambucus ebulus*), suggests using the root, leaves, stalks, and berries for dropsy (now known as edema), snakebites, burns, and coloring

---

6   Rosalee de la Forêt cites Bernard Bertrand's *Sous la Protection du Sureau.* herbalremediesadvice.org /elderberry-benefits.html#Citations
     Robert J. Losey et al., "Exploring the Use of Red Elderberry (*Sambucus racemosa*) Fruit on the Southern Northwest Coast of North America," *Journal of Archaeological Science* 30, no. 6 (June 2003), 695–707.

hair.[7] Roman author and naturalist Plinius Gaius Secondus, a.k.a. Pliny the Elder (AD 23–79) included fifteen ways to use both common and dwarf elder in the section on remedies derived from forest trees in his immense *Natural History*, including as a diuretic, purgative, skin soother, and fly repellent.[8] We now know that compounds in the plant have antimicrobial, anti-inflammatory, diuretic, and laxative properties, which is why they were found effective in diverse medical situations.

In the often-copied work of Dioscorides and in popular practice, these medicinal uses for elder spread through the Roman empire and were regularly used by peoples across Europe. Sources from the Middles Ages and Renaissance record longstanding traditions of using the elder medicinally. Bartholomaeus Anglicus, a thirteenth-century Parisian scholar who wrote a precursor to the first encyclopedia, *De proprietatibus rerum* (*On the Properties of Things*), includes separate entries for dwarf elder (*Ebulo*) and common elder (*Sambuca*) in the section on trees and plants. The description of common elder enumerates its typical uses as a treatment for fever and dropsy, noting its "vertue Diuretica."[9] German scholar Conrad von Megenberg, a prolific writer of the fourteenth century (1309–1374), best known for his *Buch der Natur* (*Book of Nature*), has been credited with the first mention of elderberry juice used to resist colds.

The sixteenth and seventeenth centuries witnessed the publication of numerous books exploring the medicinal uses of plants called "herbals," which helped to disseminate information about treating illness with plant medicine more widely. The popular 1597 *Herball, or Generall Historie of Plantes* by English botanist John Gerard includes many uses of common and dwarf elder similar to those in ancient texts, such as treating swelling, gout, and as a purgative.[10]

The most sustained look at elderberry's medicinal properties was a 1633 tome devoted entirely to elderberry, Martin Blochwich's *Anatomia Sambucii* (*The Anatomie of Elder*), a translation of Italian Army doctor C. de Iryngio's work on the subject. In 230 pages (!) Blochwich enumerates how the various parts of the elder—berries, leaves, flowers, buds, bark, roots, even a fungus that

---

7   *The Herbal of Dioscorides the Greek*, pp. 729–30. cancerlynx.com/BOOKFOURROOTS.PDF

8   Pliny the Elder, *The Natural History*, John Bostock, trans. (London: Taylor and Francis, 1855), Ch. 35, "THE ELDER: FIFTEEN REMEDIES."

9   Bartholome Anglicus. Originally published in Latin, 1240. Quotation is from a 1584 translation.

10 John Gerard, *Herball, or Generall Historie of Plantes* (London: Adam Islip, Joice Norton and Richard Whitakers, 1636) 1421–24.

grows on it called "Jew's ear"—may treat maladies of the eyes, ears, nose, mouth, and throat, alleviate a wide range of digestive complaints, arthritis, and gout, and also clear up skin conditions and wounds. He thus argues, "that not undeservedly they esteem it a Panacaea, or Allheal: For what is given to others apart, experience proves together to be in the Elder."[11]

Botanist and herbalist John Parkinson (1567–1650), a founding member of the Worshipful Society of Apothecaries and apothecary to James I, included elderberry among the 3,800 medicinal plants covered in his nearly 1,700-page *Theatrum Botanicum (Theater of Plants)*, published in 1640. The "vertues" of the common elder include many similar to those described by his predecessors, using leaves, flowers, berries, bark, and root internally and externally to treat digestive complaints, fevers, water retention, and earache, among many others.[12]

Nicolas Culpeper, seventeenth-century herbalist and author of the influential and widely-used *Complete Herbal: A Comprehensive Description of Nearly All Herbs* (1652), mentions numerous uses for elder leaves, bark, shoots, roots, flowers, and berries. He suggests them as remedies for snake and dog bites, menstrual irregularities, dropsy, ear pain, headache, bloodshot eyes, and palsies. Culpeper's herbal remained a popular source of information on herbal remedies for over a century. In Culpeper we find one of the earlier descriptions of something like an elderberry syrup, called a "Rob of Elder Berries," made from the ripe berries of either the common elder or the dwarf elder. He recommends it for dropsy: "Both Rob of Elder Berries, and Dwarf-Elder, are excellent for such whose bodies are inclining to dropsies, neither let them neglect nor despise it. They may take the quantity of a nutmeg each morning, it will gently purge the watery humour."[13]

William Coles, in his 1657 *Adam in Eden, or, Nature's Paradise: the history of plants, fruits, herbs and flowers* records many of the same uses, but stops from enumerating all of them, he says, because "should I give you all the *Vertues* of *Elder* at large, I should much exceed the usual Limits of a Chapter." He explains,

11 Martin Blochwitz. *Anatomia sambuci, or, The Anatomy of the Elder: Cutting out of it Plain, Approved, and Specific Remedies for most and chiefest Maladies ; Confirmed and cleared By Reason, Experience, and History* (London: H. Brome, 1677), 8.

12 John Parkinson, *Theatrum Botanicum: The Theater of Plants. Or, an Herbal of Large Extent* (London, Th. Cotes, 1640), 210.

13 Nicolas Culpeper, *Complete Herbal: A Comprehensive Description of Nearly All Herbs* (London: Thomas Kelly, 1801) 312.

There is hardly a *Disease*, from the *Head* to the *Foot*, but it cures; for besides the Vertues I have allready mentioned, it is profitable for the Head-Ach, for *Ravings* and *Wakings*, *Hypochondriack Mellancholy*, the *Falling-sickness*, the *Apopolexy* and *Palsy*, *Catarrhes*, *Tooth-ach*, *Deafnesse*, want of smelling, *Blemishes* of the *Face* and *Head*, *Diseases* of the *mouth* and *Throat*, the *infirmities* of the *Lungs*, *Hoasting*, and *Hoarsenesse*, the *Pleurisy* and *Ptisick*, *Women's brests being sore, swooning* and *Faintness* in *Feavours*, the *Plague*, *Pox*, *Measles*, *Diseases* of the *Stomack*, the *Wormes* and other Diseases of the *Gutts*, the *Hemorrhoides*, the *Stone*, *Diseases* of the *Matrix*, &c.[14]

Coles lists a number of ways to prepare the many useful parts of the elder—berries, flowers, roots, leaves, pith, and so on—and refers readers curious for more detail to Blochwich's *Anatomie of the Elder*. In his 1664 *Sylva: Or, a Discourse of Forest Trees & the Propagation of Timber*, John Evelyn concurs, noting the elder "is a kind of catholicon against all infirmities whatever . . . every part of the tree being useful."[15] While these claims may stretch the bounds of credulity, modern science helps to explain why elderberry appeared to address so many diverse diseases. As you'll read, the active compounds in various parts of the plant have strong antiviral activity as well as diuretic, anti-inflammatory, and laxative properties. Some research also bears out their uses against bacterial pathogens, helping to explain why they were considered useful in wound treatment, toothache, and even plague.[16]

The medicinal uses for different parts of the elder indicated by these popular herbals continued well into the nineteenth century, even as the professionalization of medicine began relegating herbal treatments to the

---

14 William Coles, *Adam in Eden, or, Nature's Paradise: the history of plants, fruits, herbs and flowers* (London: J. Streater, 1657), 297.

15 John Evelyn, *Sylva: Or, a Discourse of Forest Trees & the Propagation of Timber* (Orig. Pub 1662; reprint edition London: Doubleday, 1908), 197.

16 H. Chen et al., "Antinociceptive and Antibacterial Properties of Anthocyanins and Flavonols from Fruits of Black and Non-Black Mulberries." *Molecules* 23, no.1 (Dec 21, 2017): 4.

W. R. Yao et al. "Assessment of the Antibacterial Activity and the Antidiarrheal Function of Flavonoids from Bayberry Fruit." *Journal of Agriculture and Food Chemistry* 59, no. 10 (May 25, 2011): 5312–7.

Christian Krawitz et al., "Inhibitory Activity of a Standardized Elderberry Liquid Extract Against Clinically-Relevant Human Respiratory Bacterial Pathogens and Influenza A and B Viruses" *BMC Complementary and Alternative Medicine* 11 (2011): 16.

sidelines. John Hatfield's 1886 *Botanic Pharmacopoeia* reports that in his time elderflowers "find their principal employment in external applications, as for fomentations and poultices to swellings, and in the earlier stages of gatherings, boils, and abscesses."[17] In his 1895 *Herbal Simples Approved for Modern Uses of Cure*, William Thomas Fernie recommends numerous traditional uses of elder berries, flowers, leaves, and root for common health complaints.[18] In her 1903 *Book of Herbs*, Lady Rosalind Northcote writes, "Elder, beloved by all herbalists, still keeps its place in the British Pharmacopoeia, and the cooling effects of Elder-Flower Water, none can deny. In the country, Elder leaves and buds are most highly valued and are used in drinks, poultices, and ointments."[19]

During the first World War, British herbalist Maud Grieve transformed her plant nursery into a medicinal herb farm to help address the wartime shortage of critical medicines. In ensuing years, she devoted much of her life to herbal research, producing hundreds of monographs on medicinal plants. The monographs were collected in 1931 in a volume titled *A Modern Herbal: The Medicinal, Culinary, Cosmetic and Economic Properties, Cultivation and Folk-lore of Herbs, Grasses, Fungi, Shrubs, & Trees with All Their Modern Scientific Uses.*[20] In her lengthy section on elder's medicinal properties, she begins, "Its uses are manifold and important." She reports that the berries were used for treating rheumatism, erysipelas, bronchitis, colic, and diarrhea, and:

> Elderberry Wine has a curative power of established repute as a remedy, taken hot, at night, for promoting perspiration in the early stages of severe catarrh, accompanied by shivering, sore throat, etc. Like Elderflower Tea, it is one of the best preventives known against the advance of influenza and the ill effects of a chill . . . It has also a reputation as an excellent remedy for asthma.

17   John Hatfield, *Botanic Pharmacopoeia* (Birmingham: White and Pike 1886), 128.
18   William Thomas Fernie, *Herbal Simples: Approved for Modern Uses of Cure* (Bristol: John Wright, 1897), 164–71.
19   Lady Rosalind Northcote, *The Book of Herbs* (London: John Lane, 1903), 165.
20   Maud Grieve, *A Modern Herbal* [online resource] originally published 1931. botanical.com/botanical /mgmh/e/elder-04.html

She has much to say about the blossoms as well:

> The flowers were used by our forefathers in bronchial and pulmonary affections, and in scarlet fever, measles, and other eruptive diseases. An infusion of the dried flowers, Elder Flower Tea, is said to promote expectoration in pleurisy; it is gently laxative and aperient and is considered excellent for inducing free perspiration. It is a good old-fashioned remedy for colds and throat trouble, taken hot on going to bed. An almost infallible cure for an attack of influenza in its first stage is a strong infusion of dried Elder Blossoms and Peppermint. Put a handful of each in a jug, pour over them a pint and a half of boiling water, allow to steep, on the stove, for half an hour, then strain and sweeten and drink in bed as hot as possible.

She also mentions elderflower tea to treat inflammation of the eyes and "as a splendid spring medicine, to be taken every morning before breakfast for some weeks, being considered an excellent blood purifier."[21] Elderflowers are also recommended for external use to soothe inflammation and as a popular skin enhancer. "Elderflower Water in our great-grandmothers' days," Grieve writes, "was a household word for clearing the complexion of freckles and sunburn, and keeping it in a good condition." An official preparation in the British Pharmacopoeia known as *Aqua Sambuci*, Grieve writes, "Elder Flower Water is employed in mixing medicines and chiefly as a vehicle for eye and skin lotions," where its emollient and antimicrobial properties were especially useful.

ELDERBERRY IN NORTH AMERICA

Settlers of early America recognized the similarity of *Sambucus canadensis* to the elder plant they'd relied on in Europe, and they likewise turned to it for a variety of culinary and medicinal purposes. Native Americans had long used the American elder in ways similar to those described by European writers like Blochwich and may have shared their practices with European settlers.

---

21 Herbalist David Hoffman explains this old-fashioned term was a way to describe an "alterative," which helps organs such as the kidneys or liver to eliminate waste. David Hoffman, *The Herbal Handbook: A User's Guide to Medical Herbalism,* (VT: Healing Arts Press, 1998), 23.

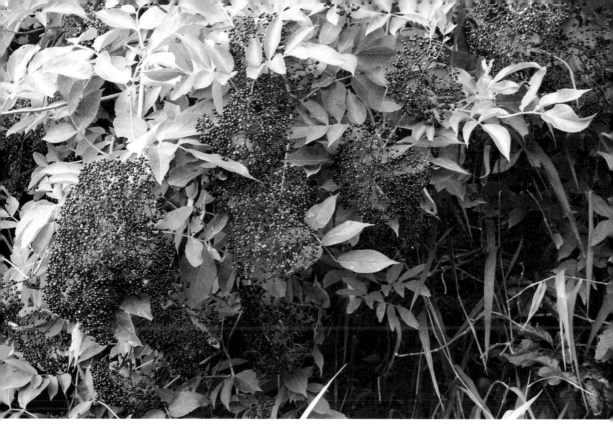

The Native American Ethnobotany Database includes hundreds of uses by tribes across the continent, including Cherokee, Iroquois, Chippewa, Dakota, Seminole and numerous others in the United States and Canada. Native Americans' uses for local varieties of elderberry (blue, black, and red) have been recorded by ethnobotanists to treat fever, skin conditions, sprains, bruises, digestive issues, rheumatism, respiratory conditions, venereal disease, toothache, and infections in both humans and animals.[22] Daniel Moerman's encyclopedic *Native American Ethnobotany* lists scores of medicinal uses, ranging from the Delaware's use of elderflower infusion for infant colic and the Cahuilla for toothache to the Choctaw's use of the root for dyspepsia. Some parts were used as emetics, while other parts had varied culinary uses, from wine and tea to cakes and pies. Moerman also records a number of tribes that made arrow shafts and bows from elder wood as well as musical instruments and children's toys.[23]

---

22 Native American Ethnobotany Database naeb.brit.org/uses/search/?string=elderberry
23 Daniel E. Moerman, *Native American Medicinal Plants: An Ethnobotanical Dictionary* (Portland, Or: Timber Press, 2009), 511–515.

European settlers of North America made frequent use of elderberry and elderflower for food and medicine, relying on herbals like Culpeper's to treat common illnesses at a time when doctors were few and far between. German-American Christopher Sauer, a printer and apothecary in Germantown, Pennsylvania, issued a series of herbal remedies in his popular German-language almanac over the course of its nearly forty-year run from 1739–1778. His discussion of elderberry includes uses for blossoms, berries, bark, pith, and leaves both internally and externally. He reportedly recommended that his readers plant elderberry bushes, which, according to an old German saying, was a "farmer's pharmacy" (*"Bauernapotheke"*).[24]

Lydia Maria Child's immensely popular 1829 *The American Frugal Housewife*—which went through thirty-three printings in twenty-five years—recommends steeping the buds of elderflowers in butter or lard to "make a very cooling and healing ointment." She also mentions "elder-blow tea," which "is cool and soothing, and peculiarly efficacious either for babes or grown people when the digestive powers are out of order."[25]

The 1845 *Quaker Woman's Cookbook*, which includes recipes in use from the earliest days of settlement, has a recipe for elderberry wine that author Elizabeth Ellicott Lea describes as "excellent as a medicine for delicate or elderly persons." She also recommends a simple tincture of elderberries and cloves as "good to give children that have the summer disease."[26] The 1849 *New England Popular Medicine* notes the widespread medicinal uses of elder, maintaining that "All good nurses in the country know the virtues of elder."[27] The 1851 *Dispensatory of the United States of America* includes elderflower water and ointment in its official preparations.[28]

During the American Civil War, army doctors used elder leaves, as well as infusions and ointments made from them, to repel flies from wounds, while infusions of elderflowers served as eyewashes and fever treatments. The inner bark was used

---

24 Christopher Sauer, *Sauer's Herbal Cures: America's First Book of Herbal Healing 1762–1778*. Translated and edited by William Woys Weaver (New York: Routledge, 2001), 129–32.

25 Lydia Maria Child, *The American Frugal Housewife* (New York: Samuel & William Wood, 1838), 29, 37.

26 Elizabeth Ellicott Lea, *Quaker Woman's Cookbook*, William Woys Weaver, ed. (Philadelphia: University of Pennsylvania Press, 1982), 151.

27 George Capron, *New England Popular Medicine: A work in which the principles and practice of medicine are familiarly explained: designed for the use of families in all parts of the United States* (Boston: George Curtis, 1849), 218.

28 George B. Wood and Franklin Bache, *Dispensatory of the United States of America* (Philadelphia : Lippincott, 1851), 646.

as an emetic and treatment for skin problems and dropsy, as described in the seventeenth-century European herbals.[29] Later in the century, American medical texts would include many of these uses, including multiple editions of *The Dispensatory of the United States of America.*[30] The 1895 *Cottage Physician* recommends elderflower in combination with a number of other ingredients for a variety of skin conditions, joint pain, "gravel and stone," measles, and inflammation of the liver.[31]

Even as modern pharmaceuticals rose to the forefront of medicine in the early twentieth century, many physicians continued to promote the value of herbal medicines like elder and used them in their practice. Doctors allied with a branch of American medicine called the Eclectic School employed both European and Native American herbalist knowledge in their treatment of illness. The nineteenth edition of *King's American Dispensatory* (1905) includes many of the historical uses listed above, as does Harvey Wickes Felter's 1922 *American Materia Medica.*[32] Dr. Edward Shook's 1946 *Advanced Treatise in Herbology* recommends cold elderflower infusion used externally for inflamed eyes, sprains, bruises, swollen glands, muscle soreness, and arthritis pain. He finds the leaves' action internally too extreme, but writes that "The leaves are, however, extremely valuable made into salves or oils for outward applications to wounds, burns, sunburn, bruises, contusions, sprains," as well as sores and many other skin conditions.[33]

I could go on. Many more herbals, pharmacopeias, and household manuals mention uses for elder, but you've probably gotten the picture by now! The next chapter, which covers scientific studies of elderberry, explores the chemical compounds researchers have identified that help to explain why these remedies worked in the days before pharmaceuticals.

People have been rediscovering the power of elderberry thanks to the explosion of interest in food-based medicine and the informative herbal and natural living websites sharing recipes and enthusiasm for elderberry-based remedies. You'll find several in the recipe section.

---

29 Cited in The Herb Society of America's "Essential Guide to Elderberry." herbsociety.org/file_download /inline/a54e481a-e368-4414-af68-2e3d42bc0bec.

30 *The Dispensatory of the United States of America*, Twelfth ed. (Philadelphia: Lippincott, 1888), 1370–1.

31 Thomas Faulkner and John Carmichael, *Cottage Physician: best known methods of treatment in all diseases, accidents and emergencies of the home* (Springfield, Mass. : King, Richardson & Co., 1892).

32 *King's American Dispensatory* (Cincinnati: Ohio Valley Company, 1905), 1706–8.
     Harvey Wickes Felter, *American Materia Medica* (1922) henriettes-herb.com/eclectic/felter /sambucus.html.

33 Quoted in Wood, pp 432–3.

ELDER LORE

In addition to its many medicinal uses, and perhaps because of them, the elder tree inspired a rich folklore that invested the plant with strong magical powers. One legend had it that Christ's cross was made from elder wood, while in another Judas hung himself from an elder tree. A common Scottish rhyme tells us that since the crucifixion, the elder (bour-tree) changed in form:

> Bour-tree, Bour-tree, crooked rung,
> Never straight and never strong,
> Ever bush and never tree,
> Since our Lord was nailed on thee.[34]

These legends likely inspired the many connections of elder with forces of evil. In England and Scandinavia, woodsmen asked permission before cutting elders or risked arousing the wrath of the dryad Hyldemoer (Elder Mother), a sometime goddess of plants, sometime witch believed to inhabit elder trees. A Celtic rhyme reminds us, "Elder be ye Lady's tree, burn it not or cursed ye'll be."

In *The Folklore of Plants*, T. F. Thiselton-Dyer relates that "The elder tree is another haunt under whose branches witches are fond of lurking, and on this account caution must be taken not to tamper with it after dark."[35] In *Plant Lore: Legends and Lyrics*, Richard Folkard explains, "the Elder appears to have invariably possessed a certain weird attraction for mischievous Elves and Witches, who are fond of seeking the shelter of its pendent boughs, and are wont to bury their satanic offspring, with certain cabalistic ceremonies, beneath its roots."[36] In *The Book of Herbs*, Lady Northcote remarks, "Every inch of an Elder-tree is connected with magic." In Danish folklore, for example, "if furniture is made of the wood, Hylde-Moer may follow her property and haunt and worry the owners, and there is a tradition that once when a child was put in a cradle of Elder-wood, Hylde-Moer came and pulled it by the legs and would give it no peace till it was lifted out."[37]

---

34   Richard Folkard, *Plant Lore: Legends and Lyrics* (London: Folkard & Son, 1884), 321.
35   Thomas Firminger Thiselton-Dyer, *The Folk-lore of Plants* (London: Chatto & Windus, 1889), 58.
36   Folkard, 92.
37   Northcote, 183–4.

However, the elder was also thought powerfully protective. Thiselton-Dyer explains:

> According to an old tradition, any baptized person whose eyes were anointed with the green juice of its inner bark could see witches in any part of the world. Hence the tree was extremely obnoxious to witches, a fact which probably accounts for its having so often been planted near cottages. Its magic influence has also caused it to be introduced into various rites, as in Styria on Bertha Night (January 6th), when the devil goes about in great force. As a safeguard, persons are recommended to make a magic circle, in the centre of which they should stand with elder-berries gathered on St. John's night.[38]

A number of historical sources mention the tradition that elder leaves "gathered on the last day of April, and affixed to the doors and windows of the house, disappoints designing Witches and protects the inhabitants from their diabolical spells."[39] In several European countries, April 30 is known as Walpurgis night, celebrating Saint Walpurga, a Christian missionary noted for her work combating both disease and witchcraft.

While the flowers were sometimes used to make an antiseptic mouth rinse, the Danes sought to harness the magic powers of the plant to treat dental woes. Thiselton-Dyer explains that "a Danish cure for toothache consists in placing an elder-twig in the mouth, and then sticking it in a wall, saying, 'Depart, thou evil spirit.'"[40] Compounds in the wood may have had an antiseptic effect on infected teeth, making this a doubly powerful treatment. Whether for its medicinal or its magical properties, the Danes valued elder highly, hence the Danish proverb "Where the elder won't grow, man cannot live."

Elder's power to ward off evil and bad luck led to several traditions of planting it near homes and gardens to protect them. In the Middle Ages leaves were placed around buildings to keep away spirits. William Thomas Fernie relates that "Formerly it was much cultivated near our English cottages, because supposed to afford protection against witches. Hence it is that the Elder tree may be so often seen immediately near old village houses." Elder was also thought

---

38 Thiselton-Dyer, 75.
39 Folkard, 103.
40 Thiselton-Dyer, 288.

lightning-proof, he explains, and "at the present day a person is said to be perfectly safe under an elder tree during a thunderstorm."[41]

Lady Northcote's research yielded similar traditions in other parts of Europe:

> The Russians believe that Elder-trees drive away evil spirits, and the Bohemians go to it with a spell to take away fever. The Sicilians think that sticks of its wood will kill serpents and drive away robbers, and the Serbs introduce a stick of Elder into their wedding ceremonies to bring good luck. In England it was thought that the Elder was never struck by lightning, and a twig of it tied into three or four knots and carried in the pocket was a charm against rheumatism. A cross made of Elder and fastened to cowhouses and stables was supposed to keep all evil from the animals.[42]

Legend had it that the elder shrub served as a gateway to the underworld, giving rise to its use in rituals surrounding burials. Grieve relates a tradition in Austria in which "'An Elder bush, trimmed into the form of a cross, is planted on a new-made grave, and if it blossoms, the soul of the person lying beneath it is happy.'" Additionally, she says, "Green Elder branches were also buried in a grave to protect the dead from witches and evil spirits, and in some parts it was a custom for the driver of the hearse to carry a whip made of Elder wood."

The ELDER FLOWER Fairy

The Elder Fairy, Cicely Mary Barker, c.1923

Elder lore connected this powerful plant with fairies and magical realms. Lady Northcote recounts a tradition that "He who stands under an Elder-tree at midnight on Midsummer Eve may chance to see Toly, the King of Elves, and all his retinue go by."[43] A similar tradition appears in Scottish folklore. Maud Grieve suggests this legend may have arisen because of the "narcotic smell" the elder emits, noting that "it is not considered wise to sleep under its shade. Perhaps the visions of fairyland were the result of the drugged sleep!"

---

41 Fernie, 170.
42 Northcote, 184.
43 Northcote, 184.

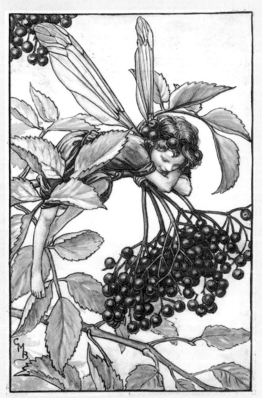

The Elderberry Fairy, Cicely Mary Barker, 1923

Popular nineteenth-century Danish author Hans Christian Andersen featured the magical elder in several of his fairy tales. It figures most prominently in his 1844 story "The Elder-Tree Mother," in which a little boy, having gotten his feet wet and caught cold, is served "a good cup of elder tea" by his mother to warm him. A fantastic adventure ensues:

And the little boy looked toward the teapot. He saw the lid slowly raise itself and fresh white elder flowers come forth from it. They shot long branches even out of the spout and spread them abroad in all directions, and they grew bigger and bigger until there was the most glorious elder bush—really a big tree! The branches even stretched to the little boy's bed and thrust the curtains aside—how fragrant its blossoms were! And right in the middle of the tree there sat a sweet-looking old woman in a very strange dress. It was green, as green as the leaves of the elder tree, and it was trimmed with big white elder blossoms; at first, one couldn't tell if this dress was cloth or the living green and flowers of the tree.

"What is this woman's name?" asked the little boy.

"Well, the Romans and the Greeks," said the old man, "used to call her a 'Dryad,' but we don't understand that word. Out in New Town, where the sailors live, they have a better name for her. There she is called 'Elder Tree Mother,' and you must pay attention to her; listen to her, and look at that glorious elder tree![44]

44 Hans Christian Andersen, "The Elder-Tree Mother," in *Hans Christian Andersen's Complete Fairy Tales*, trans. Jean Hershort. (San Diego, Canterbury Classics, 2014), 198–203.

The little boy dreams that the Elder-Tree Mother takes him from his bed and flies with him through space and time with "the blooming branches of elder closed over them so that they sat, as it were, in a leafy bower, and the bower flew with them through the air in the most delight-ful manner." She shows him distant places and times, eventually revealing that her "real name is Memory." When he wakes, he finds the Elder-Tree Mother has returned to the teapot, but "there were thousands of pic-tures in the boy's mind and heart."

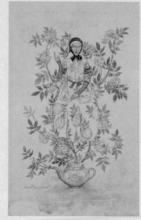

The Elder Mother, Arthur Rackham, 1932.

OTHER TIDBITS OF ELDERBERRY TRIVIA:

One of elder's more common forms in Europe and the United States was wine made from elderberries, sometimes consumed medicinally, but also simply as wine. When made well, many writers compared elderberry wine favorably to fine ports and frontignac, but I've been told by elderberry growers it's not easy to make well, so often wasn't very tasty. An ailing Walt Whitman reportedly served some made by his sister-in-law Louisa to the young aesthete Oscar Wilde when he visited the United States in 1882. J. M. Stoddart, Wilde's publisher, joined the two and recalled to a journalist some years later, "After we were seated he brought out some elderberry wine which tasted vile beyond description. Wilde drank two or three glasses with evident relish and when we left I asked him how he liked it. 'It was poor stuff,' he said, 'but I would have drank it had it been vinegar.'"[45]

The tradition of home brewing elderberry wine carried on into the twenti-eth century (and beyond—if you'd like to try it yourself, you'll find a recipe on page 166). In the 1939 play *Arsenic and Old Lace* (made into the well-known 1944 film starring Cary Grant), two maiden aunts famously murder their lodgers with elderberry wine laced with arsenic and other poisons. Elton John's 1972 hit "Elderberry Wine," reminisces about "feeling fine on elderberry wine," while the Rolling Stones 1974 song "Till the Next Goodbye" laments, "Some cider vinegar and some elderberry wine/ May cure all your ills, but it can't cure mine."

---

45 *Kansas City Journal*, November 12, 1899, 12. Oscar Wilde in America oscarwildeinamerica.org /features/wilde-meets-whitman.html.

If you mention that you're using elderberries in earshot of any Monty Python fan, they will surely quote (or misquote) one of the more famous exchanges from the 1975 film *Monty Python and the Holy Grail*. If you haven't seen it, be sure to check out the hilarious string of insults hurled by the French castle guard that winds up with "Your mother was a hamster and your father smelt of elderberries!"

Elderberry saw a notable uptick in reputation when J. K. Rowling chose elder as the wood for the most powerful wand ever made in her final Harry Potter book, *The Deathly Hallows*, which she considered titling *The Elder Wand*. [46]

The elder wand is just one of many crafts made from elder wood, which because of its hollow center, has been a popular choice across the centuries for children's toys like popguns and whistles. Maud Grieve recounts a number of common uses for elder wood:

> The wood of old trees is white and of a fine, close grain, easily cut, and polishes well, hence it was used for making skewers for butchers, shoe-makers' pegs, and various turned articles, such as tops for angling rods and needles for weaving nets, also for making combs, mathematical instruments and several different musical instruments, and the pith of the younger stems, which is exceedingly light, is cut into balls and is used for electrical experiments and for making small toys. It is also considerably used for holding small objects for sectioning for microscopical purposes.

It was also used by Native Americans for making arrows, fire-blowing tubes, and ceremonial objects.

The juice from the berries—which stains everything it touches—has also been used as a food and clothing dye, and is one of the ingredients used in dyes for inspection stamps on meat. Elderberry-based ink was used in the American Civil War, and according to Rosalee de la Forêt, by French school children until quite recently. I found some instructions on making inks from berries and include a recipe on page 180 if you want to try it for yourself.

Now that you're well versed in elderberry's colorful history, let's move on to how you can use it today.

---

46 Transcript of JK Rowling web chat, HPANA hpana.com/news/20137.

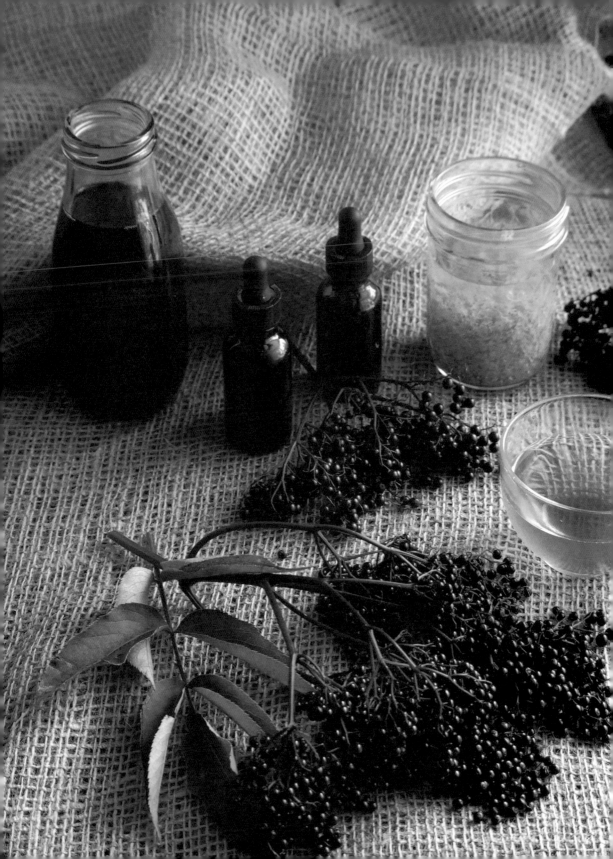

CHAPTER 2

USING ELDERBERRY TO PROMOTE HEALTH

"But if the medicinal properties of the leaves, bark, berries, &c. were thoroughly known, I cannot tell what our countrey-man could ail, for which he might not fetch a remedy from every hedge, either for sickness or wound."
—John Evelyn, *Sylva* (1664)[1]

While some of the accolades for elderberries' medicinal uses may seem quaintly far-fetched, the idea that preparations made from this plant can treat a wide range of illnesses might not be as improbable as it seems. Biochemists studying the key constituents of the elderberry's fruit, leaves, bark, and flowers have discovered they indeed have a broad range of effects that include reducing inflammation, interfering with viral activity, and promoting circulatory health.

Scientific Research on Elderberry

Elderberries' recent surge in popularity can be largely attributed to the numerous scientific studies suggesting their legendary ability to fight infection may have merit. To date, hundreds of studies have investigated the chemical composition, biological activity, and health effects of elderberries and elderflowers. However, only a fraction of these studies were conducted on human subjects, and most of those used small numbers of participants, so further research is required to fulfill the stringent requirements for scientific validity. Other researchers have conducted experiments on rodents, but since humans and rodents don't necessarily respond in the same way, our ability to extrapolate from these studies is limited. Numerous other studies examined the action of elderberry *in vitro* (on cells in a lab rather than in live subjects), which can tell us a little about the chemical and biological activity of elder's compounds, but not how they will work in the human body when ingested or applied to the skin. Complicating our understanding of herbal medicine's efficacy, herbalist Rosalee de la Forêt points out, many studies investigating the actions of herbal

---

1   Evelyn, 197.

remedies are designed with little regard to traditional preparation and dosing, often using what she views as far too little of the herb or with insufficient frequency or duration.

Researchers continue to seek answers about how the biologically-active constituents in elderberries actually work in our bodies. Search the National Institutes of Health's PubMed database for "sambucus," and you'll find over a thousand studies. The majority use compounds isolated from elderberries on cells *in vitro* to examine how those compounds affect different types of cells and microbes. Peter Valtchev, who co-authored a 2019 study looking at elderberry's anti-influenza activity, explained to me that *in vitro* studies like his were primarily "useful for determining the mechanism of activity," which can help pinpoint the compounds involved in the herb's action. In vitro studies don't, however, tell us anything about how the compounds in elderberries behave in our bodies after we metabolize them.

So what do we know about how elderberry works? Though that is still a matter of debate, elderberries contain a number of compounds widely believed to support health in a variety of ways. Elderberries contain high concentrations of compounds called flavonoids, which are prized for their ability to combat what's known as "oxidative stress," a state in which our bodies have an excess of unstable atoms called free radicals. Free radicals can damage DNA, cells, and proteins, leading to health consequences that include the development of cancer, neurological diseases, and inflammatory conditions like arthritis. All kinds of normal bodily processes produce free radicals, but things hard to avoid in the modern world, like air pollution and exposures to chemicals in the environment and food supply, can increase how many we produce, with damaging effects. Psychological stress, lack of sleep, smoking, and a diet high in processed foods and sugar have also been linked to oxidative stress.

Put simply, if we can keep our levels of free radicals in check, we may stand a better chance of avoiding many of these diseases. Enter antioxidants, like those we find in elderberries and elderflowers, which scientists believe protect us from oxidative stress by countering free radicals.[2] Dark berries have high con-

---

2   V. Lobo et al., "Free radicals, Antioxidants and Functional foods: Impact on Human health," *Pharmacognosy Review* 4, no.8 (Jul-Dec 2010): 118–126. J. K. Willcox et al., "Antioxidants and Prevention of Chronic Disease," *Critical Reviews in Food Science and Nutrition* 44, no. 4 (2004): 275–95. Karel Cejpek et al., "Antioxidant Activity in Variously Prepared Elderberry Foods and Supplements." *Czech Journal of Food Sciences* 27, Special Issue 1 (January 2009).

centrations of antioxidants, and elderberries are an exceptionally rich source.[3] A 2015 review of human studies of elderberry noted that the compounds in elderberries "can greatly affect the course of disease processes by counteracting oxidative stress, exerting beneficial effects on blood pressure, glycaemia reduction, immune system stimulation, anti-tumour potential, increase in the activity of antioxidant enzymes in the blood plasma."[4] Analyses of the antioxidants in elderflowers suggest that levels exceed those found in elderberries.[5] One well-studied antioxidant found in elderberries, anthocyanin, has been found to reduce inflammation, a key player in the development of common chronic diseases. Numerous studies have looked at the anti-inflammatory effects of anthocyanins, which help to promote heart, brain, and metabolic health and seem to lower risk of many diseases, including cancer.[6]

ELDERBERRY'S ANTIVIRAL ACTION

Emerging research indicates that compounds in elderberry interfere with viral replication, helping to shorten the duration and severity of flu. Lab studies suggest that elderberry may both stimulate the body's response to infection and inhibit viruses' ability to penetrate host cells. A 2019 study found that elderberry extract had multiple antiviral actions, blocking viruses from infecting cells, interfering with viral replication in infected cells, and stimulating the production of

3   A. Viapiana et al., "The Phenolic Contents and Antioxidant Activities of Infusions of Sambucus nigra L.," *Plant Foods for Human Nutrition* 72, no. 1 (March 2017): 82–87.
    Kuresh Youdim et al., "Incorporation of the Elderberry Anthocyanins by Endothelial Cells Increases Protection Against Oxidative Stress," *Free Radical Biology and Medicine* 29, no. 1, (July 2000): 51–60.

4   Andrzej Sidor and Anna Gramza-Michałowska, "Advanced research on the antioxidant and health benefit of elderberry (Sambucus nigra) in food – a review," *Journal of Functional Foods* 18, part B (October 2015): 941–958.

5   Karolina Młynarczyk et al., "Bioactive Properties of *Sambucus nigra* L. as a Functional Ingredient for Food and Pharmaceutical Industry," *Journal of Functional Foods* 40 (January 2018): 377–390.

6   Yoon-Mi Lee et al., "Dietary Anthocyanins against Obesity and Inflammation," *Nutrients* 9, no. 10 (October 2017).
    Arpita Basu, "Berries: Emerging Impact on Cardiovascular Health," *Nutrition Review* 68, no. 3 (March 2010): 168–177.
    Aedín Cassidy et al., "High Anthocyanin Intake Is Associated With a Reduced Risk of Myocardial Infarction in Young and Middle-Aged Women," *Circulation* 127, no. 2 (January 2013): 188–196.
    Y. He et al., "Antioxidant and Anti-inflammatory Effects of Cyanidin from Cherries on Rat Adjuvant-Induced Arthritis," *Zhongguo Zhong Yao Za Zhi* 30, no. 20 (October 2005): 1602–5.

cytokines, chemical messengers that coordinate our immune response.[7] One *in vitro* experiment found flavonoids from elderberry extract blocked infection by the H1N1 flu virus as effectively as the flu medication Tamiflu.[8]

Some early studies on human subjects conducted in Israel in the 1990s found treatment with the elderberry syrup now sold as Sambucol® significantly reduced the duration of flu symptoms, prompting researchers around the world to conduct studies of their own.[9] In 2004, Norwegian researchers published a study of sixty subjects, finding that "Symptoms were relieved on average 4 days earlier and use of rescue medication was significantly less in those receiving elderberry extract compared with placebo" in patients with two strains of flu.[10] A 2009 Chinese study of sixty-four patients with flu-like symptoms found that "elderberry extract can rapidly relieve influenza-like symptoms . . . While the placebo group demonstrated no symptoms improvement, the proprietary elderberry extract treated group showed significant improvement of influenza-like symptoms within 24 hours of the onset of treatment."[11]

A 2016 study of more than 300 Australian air travelers found a significant reduction in duration and reported severity of colds in the group that supplemented with elderberry versus the group given a placebo. Participants took capsules containing elderberry extract or a placebo before and during their trip and kept a diary of cold symptoms. Though roughly the same number of people in each group caught colds, those who took elderberry had significantly fewer days with cold symptoms.[12]

A 2019 metastudy reviewing the extant research on elderberry concluded, "Supplementation with elderberry was found to substantially reduce upper

7   Golnoosh Torabian et al., "Anti-influenza Activity of Elderberry (*Sambucus nigra*)," *Journal of Functional Foods* 54 (March 2019): 353–60.
8   Bill Roschek Jr. et al., "Elderberry Flavonoids Bind to and Prevent H1N1 Infection *in Vitro*," *Phytochemistry* 70, no. 10 (July 2009): 1255–61.
9   Zichria Zakay-Rones et al., "Inhibition of Several Strains of Influenza Virus in Vitro and Reduction of Symptoms by an Elderberry Extract (*Sambucus nigra* L.) During an Outbreak of Influenza B Panama," *The Journal of Alternative and Complementary Medicine* 1, No. 4 (Winter 1995): 361–9.
10 Zichria Zakay-Rones et al., "Randomized Study of the Efficacy and Safety of Oral Elderberry Extract in the Treatment of Influenza A and B Virus Infections," *Journal International Medical Research* 32, no. 2 (March-April 2004): 132–40.
11 Fan-kun Kong, "Pilot Clinical Study on a Proprietary Elderberry Extract: Efficacy in Addressing Influenza Symptoms." *Online Journal of Pharmacology and PharmacoKinetics* 5 (2009): 32–43.
12 Evelin Tiralongo et al., "Elderberry Supplementation Reduces Cold Duration and Symptoms in Air-Travellers: A Randomized, Double-Blind Placebo-Controlled Clinical Trial," *Nutrients* 8, no. 4 (April 2016): 182.

respiratory symptoms," especially in cases of flu, and to a lesser extent with colds. "The effect of elderberry supplementation is larger among cases of the flu than the common cold," study authors determined, "but supplementation successfully reduces the symptoms regardless of underlying cause."[13]

Some of elderberry's impact on colds and flu may come from its antioxidants' protective effect on tissues in the respiratory system. Anthocyanins have been detected in lung tissue shortly after consumption, and a 2016 analysis of participants in the VA Normative Aging Study reported that "strong inverse associations were found between anthocyanin intake and age-related decline in lung function."[14] A 2018 epidemiological study also found that participants with the highest consumption of anthocyanins in the European Community Health Survey had better measures of lung health.[15]

Elderberry's antiviral activity has also prompted researchers to investigate its usefulness against HIV.[16]

EFFECTS ON THE CIRCULATORY SYSTEM

Anthocyanins' anti-inflammatory effects have spurred research into elderberries' effect on a number of health conditions related to inflammation, including cardiovascular disease. Foods rich in anthocyanins appear to have "significant beneficial effects in vascular disease," while population studies suggest that diets high in flavonoids like anthocyanin "significantly decrease the risk of CVD [cardiovascular disease]."[17] One study found that rats given elderberry extract

---

13 Jessie Hawkins et al., "Black elderberry (*Sambucus nigra*) Supplementation Effectively Treats Upper Respiratory Symptoms: A Meta-Analysis of Randomized, Controlled Clinical Trials," *Complementary Therapies in Medicine* 42 (February 2019): 361–365.

14 Amar J Mehta et al., "Dietary Anthocyanin Intake and Age-Related Decline in Lung Function: Longitudinal Findings from the VA Normative Aging Study." *American Journal of Clinical Nutrition* 103, no. 2 (2016 Feb): 542–550.

15 V. Garcia Larsen et al., "Dietary Intake of Anthocyanin Flavonoids and Ten Year Lung Function Decline in Adults from the European Community Respiratory Health Survey (ECRHS) *American Journal of Respiratory and Critical Care Medicine* 197 (2018): A2797.

16 R. E. Uncini Manganelli et al., "Antiviral Activity in vitro of *Urtica dioica* L., *Parietaria diffusa* M. et K. and *Sambucus nigra* L." *Journal of Ethnopharmacology* 98, no. 3 (April 26, 2005): 323–7.

17 X. Wang et al., "Flavonoid Intake and Risk of CVD: A Systematic Review and Meta-Analysis of Prospective Cohort Studies," *British Journal of Nutrition* 111, no. 1 (January 14, 2014): 1–11. However, one study found that elderberry extract did not relax coronary arteries. David R. Bell, and Kristen Gochenaur, "Direct vasoactive and vasoprotective properties of anthocyanin-rich extracts," *Journal of Applied Physiology* 100, No. 4 (April 2006): 1164–1170.

had reduced blood pressure,[18] though a human study using an elderberry-derived anthocyanin found no change in markers of CVD after twelve weeks.[19]

Quercetin, another compound found in elderberries, is believed to lower blood pressure and have a positive effect on cholesterol.[20] A 2015 study conducted at the University of Connecticut found significant improvement in cholesterol levels in mice fed elderberry extract.[21]

DIABETES AND METABOLISM

Both elderberry and elderflower are traditional treatments for diabetes, and emerging research bears out this centuries-old use. Several animal studies have demonstrated elderberry's positive effect on glucose levels and insulin resistance. A 2017 study found that elderberry extract lowered insulin resistance in diabetic rats.[22] Another study determined that "The antidiabetic properties found in phenolics from elderflower increase the nutritional value of this plant as a functional food against diabetes."[23]

Elderberry extract has shown promise for the treatment of other metabolic disorders as well. A 2015 animal study published in the *British Journal of Nutrition* found that elderberry extract significantly reduced inflammation and metabolic dysfunction in obese animals.[24] A 2019 *in vitro* study

---

18 M. Ciocoiu et al., "The Beneficial Effects on Blood Pressure, Dyslipidemia and Oxidative Stress of Sambucus nigra Extract Associated with Renin Inhibitors," *Pharmaceutical Biology* 54, no. 12 (December 2016): 3063–3067.
       Anca Iuliana Moroşanu et al., "Antioxidant Effect of Aronia Versus Sambucus on Murine Model with or without Arterial Hypertension," *Annals of the Romanian Society for Cell Biology* 16, no. 1 (January 2011): 222–227.
19 This experiment may have used only one isolated compound in elderberry, and other studies have found that individual constituents do not necessarily have the same effect as the whole food. Peter J. Curtis et al., "Cardiovascular Disease Risk Biomarkers and Liver and Kidney Function are Not Altered in Postmenopausal Women after Ingesting an Elderberry Extract Rich in Anthocyanins for 12 Weeks." *Journal of Nutrition* 139, no. 12 (September 2009): 2266–71.
20 Haohai Huang et al., "Effect of Quercetin Supplementation on Plasma Lipid Profiles, Blood pressure, and Glucose Levels: A Systematic Review and Meta-Analysis," *Nutrition Reviews* (January 6, 2020): nuz071.
21 Nicholas Farrell et al., "Anthocyanin-Rich Black Elderberry Extract Improves Markers of HDL Function and Reduces Aortic Cholesterol in Hyperlipidemic Mice," *Food and Function* 4 (2015): 1278–87.
22 Ângelo C. Salvador et al., "Effect of Elderberry (Sambucus nigra L.) Extract Supplementation in STZ-Induced Diabetic Rats Fed with a High-Fat Diet," *International Journal Molecular Sciences*, 18, no. 1 (January 2017): 13.
23 Giang Thanh Thi Ho et al., "Effect of Phenolic Compounds from Elderflowers on Glucose- and Fatty Acid Uptake in Human Myotubes and HepG2-Cells," *Molecules* 22, no. 1 (January 6, 2017). pii: E90.
24 N. J. Farrell et al., "Black Elderberry Extract Attenuates Inflammation and Metabolic Dysfunction in Diet-Induced Obese Mice," *British Journal of Nutrition* 114, no. 8 (August 2015): 1–9

concluded, "Sambucus nigra fruit extract may offer substantial preventive and therapeutic potential for the treatment of obesity and obesity-related disorders, accompanied by oxidative stress, inflammation, and insulin resistance."[25]

BRAIN HEALTH

You may have heard that blueberries can protect your brain from the effects of age-related decline. With an even greater concentration of brain-protective anthocyanins, whether elderberry can enhance cognitive function is another line of scientific inquiry.[26]

One animal study demonstrated that feeding rats berries high in antioxidants helped "to prevent and reverse the neurochemical and behavioral changes that occur in aging, such as loss of memory, cognition, and motor functions."[27] Another study in humans found that forty participants ages 50–70 given a drink of mixed berry extract (which included elderberry) "performed better in the working memory test after the berry beverage compared to after the control beverage," though without further research we can't be sure how much we can chalk up to elderberry.[28] Dennis Lubahn, Director of the University of Missouri's Center on Botanical Interactions Studies, told me that an unpublished study looking at elderberry's ability to protect the brain from stroke damage found that elderberry extract was "Really quite spectacular . . . in the prevention of damage from stroke."

CANCER PREVENTION AND TREATMENT

Like other antioxidant-rich foods, elderberry contains a number of compounds believed to have a protective effect against cancer, which may develop in

25 Joanna Zielińska-Wasielica et al., "Elderberry (*Sambucus nigra* L.) Fruit Extract Alleviates Oxidative Stress, Insulin Resistance, and Inflammation in Hypertrophied 3T3-L1 Adipocytes and Activated RAW 264.7 Macrophages," *Foods* 8, no. 8 (August 2019): 326.

26 Ongoing clinical trial on cognitive decline at University of Missouri: David Beversdorf, clinicaltrials .gov/ct2/show/NCT02414607

27 Shibu M. Poulose and Barbara Shukitt-Hale, "Effect of Berries on Cognitive and Neurochemical Functions," paper presented at the First International Symposium on Elderberry, 2013. centerforagroforestry .org/profit/ElderberrySymposiumGuide.pdf

28 A. Nilsson et al., "Effects of a Mixed Berry Beverage on Cognitive Functions and Cardiometabolic Risk Markers: A Randomized Cross-Over Study in Healthy Older Adults," *PLoS One* 12, no. 11 (November 15, 2017): e0188173.

response to oxidative stress.[29] A 2018 *in vitro* study found that elderberry extract demonstrated anti-cancer activity, and a 2006 analysis of compounds derived from wild and cultivated American and European varieties of elderberry determined that "Both cultivated S. nigra and wild S. canadensis fruits demonstrated significant chemopreventive potential."[30] University of Missouri researchers found that feeding mice freeze-dried elderberry juice significantly slowed the growth of prostate cancer.[31]

Ukranian scientists are investigating how compounds in elderberry plants reduce DNA damage that can lead to cancer.[32] Research suggests that consumption of foods high in antioxidants may help prevent skin cancer, and elderberries are also being studied as a topical treatment for skin cancer.[33]

VARIATION IN COMPOSITION OF BERRIES

Some research has endeavored to evaluate the amounts of these active compounds in different varieties of elderberry. Studies conducted in Slovenia found varying levels of polyphenols in different varieties and in plants grown at different elevations, while a study comparing European and American varieties found no substantive difference in the amounts of flavonoids and other

---

29 Cuiwei Zhao et al., "Effects of Commercial Anthocyanin-Rich Extracts on Colonic Cancer and Nontumorigenic Colonic Cell Growth," *Journal of Agricultural Food Chemistry* 52, no. 20 (September 14, 2004): 6122–6128.

30 Paulina Strugała et al., "A Comprehensive Study on the Biological Activity of Elderberry Extract and Cyanidin 3-*O*-Glucoside and Their Interactions with Membranes and Human Serum Albumin," *Molecules* 23, no. 10 (October 2018): 2566.

    J. Thole et al., "A Comparative Evaluation of the Anticancer Properties of European and American Elderberry fruits," *Journal of Medicinal Food* 9, no. 4 (Winter 2006): 498–504.

    A. Olejnik et al., "A Gastrointestinal Digested *Sambucus nigra* L. Fruit Extract Protects *in vitro* Cultured Human Colon Cells Against Oxidative Stress," *Food Chemistry* 197, Pt. A (Apr 15, 2016): 648–57.

31 Glenn Jackson et al., "Elderberry Juice Prevents Prostate Cancer *In Vitro* and in an *In Vivo* Mouse Model." Paper presented at The First International Symposium on Elderberry, Columbia, Missouri, 2013.

32 Iryna Karpova et al., "Lectins of *Sambucus nigra* as Biologically Active and DNA-Protective Substances," Paper presented at The First International Symposium on Elderberry, Columbia, Missouri, 2013.

33 Joi A. Nichols and Santosh K. Katiyar, "Skin Photoprotection by Natural Polyphenols: Anti-Inflammatory, Antioxidant and DNA Repair Mechanisms." *Archives of Dermatological Research* 302, no. 2 (March 2010): 71–83.

    Dumitrita Rugină et al., "Antiproliferative and Apoptotic Potential of Cyanidin-Based Anthocyanins on Melanoma Cells," *International Journal of Molecular Sciences* 18, no. 5 (April 2017): 0949.

cancer-fighting compounds.[34] Another study found that extended freezing may significantly reduce levels of anthocyanins.[35]

What does all this information mean to you, the consumer? While all the interest in the scientific community in identifying precise mechanisms of elderberry in the body shows something powerful is going on here, we probably shouldn't start worrying too much about the exact composition of our elderberries and how much or how little consuming elderberries may affect our risk of developing one disease or another. However, if you already have one of the diseases mentioned above or have a family history of one, incorporating elderberry into a varied, nutrient-rich diet may be worth discussing with your doctor. If you're generally healthy, including this dark berry in your rainbow of food choices may well help keep you that way. The burden of proof in modern science is extremely high (and very expensive), so don't expect definitive answers anytime soon. In the meantime, science suggests that enjoying a range of deeply-colored plants, including elderberry, may benefit our health in numerous ways.

Elderflower Benefits and Uses

The medicinal properties of elderflower have not received as much scientific attention as elderberry, but as we saw in the history section, elderflower has been a remedy for colds and respiratory conditions for centuries. Elderflowers are especially prized for treating fevers and seasonal allergies. Herbalist jim mcdonald writes, "The dried flowers of Elder

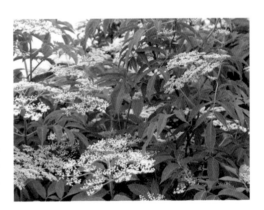

---

34 M. Mikulic-Petkovsek et al., "Fruit Phenolic Composition of Different Elderberry Species and Hybrids," *Journal of Food Science* 80, no. 10 (Oct. 2015): C2180-90.

Mateja Senica et al., "The Higher the Better? Differences in Phenolics and Cyanogenic Glycosides in *Sambucus nigra* Leaves, Flowers and Berries from Different Altitudes," *Journal of the Science of Food and Agriculture* 97, no. 8 (June 2017): 2623-32

35 M. C. Johnson et al., "Impact of Frozen Storage on the Anthocyanin and Polyphenol Contents of American Elderberry Fruit Juice." *Journal of Agricultural and Food Chemistry* 63, no. 23 (June 17, 2015): 5653-9.

are one of the oldest and most reliable diaphoretics for use in treating colds, flus & fevers."[36]

In recent years, scientists have investigated elderflower's impressive antioxidant capacity and are exploring its use as a therapy for Parkinson's disease and breast cancer as well as for controlling blood sugar and cholesterol.[37]

Externally, elderflower may offer some protection against damage from UV rays, according to one study.[38] Another *in vitro* study found elderflower extract inhibited pathogens involved in periodontitis, while additional studies found both elderflower and elderberry useful against pathogens such as MRSA.[39]

Using Elder Like an Herbalist

Though the science backing up elder's many uses for treating illness and promoting good health cannot be considered conclusive, as we saw in Chapter 1, herbalists have used different parts of the elder as medicine for hundreds of years. Modern herbalists attest to elder's value in their practice and use elderberries

---

36 jim mcdonald, "Elder." herbcraft.org/elder.html

37 Jaquet de Rus et al., "Lumbee Traditional Medicine: Neuroprotective Activities of Medicinal Plants Used to Treat Parkinson's Disease-Related Symptoms," *Journal of Ethnopharmacology* 12, no. 206 (July 2017): 408–425.
    L. Schröder et al., "Effects of Phytoestrogen Extracts Isolated from Elder Flower on Hormone Production and Receptor Expression of Trophoblast Tumor Cells JEG-3 and BeWo, as well as MCF7 Breast Cancer Cells," *Nutrients* 8, no. 10 (Oct 8, 2016): E616.
    S. Bhattacharya et al., "Bioactive Components from Flowers of Sambucus nigra L. Increase Glucose Uptake in Primary Porcine Myotube Cultures and Reduce Fat Accumulation in Caenorhabditis elegans." *Journal of Agriculture and Food Chemistry* 61, no. 46 (November 20, 2013): 11033–40.
    K. B. Christensen et al., "Identification of Bioactive Compounds from Flowers of Black Elder (Sambucus nigra L.) that Activate the Human Peroxisome Proliferator-Activated Receptor (PPAR) gamma." *Phytotherapy Research* Suppl 2 (June 24, 2010): S129-32.

38 Anna Jarzycka, et al., "Assessment of extracts of Helichrysum arenarium, Crataegus monogyna, Sambucus nigra in photoprotective UVA and UVB; photostability in cosmetic emulsions." *Journal of Photochemistry and Photobiology B: Biology* 128, 5 (November 2013): 50–57.
    J. A. Nichols and S. K. Katiyar. "Skin photoprotection by natural polyphenols: anti-inflammatory, antioxidant and DNA repair mechanisms." *Archives of Dermatological Research* 302, no. 2 (March 2010).

39 E. Harokopakis et al., "Inhibition of Proinflammatory Activities of Major Periodontal Pathogens by Aqueous Extracts from Elder Flower (Sambucus nigra**)**. *Journal of Periodontology* 77, no. 2 (February 2006): 271–9.
    Caroline Hearst et al., "Antibacterial Activity of Elder (*Sambucus nigra L.*) Flower or Berry Against Hospital Pathogens," *Journal of Medicinal Plants Research* 4, no. 17 (September 4, 2010): pp. 1805–1809.
    Claudio Andrés Álvarez et al., "Identification of Peptides in Flowers of Sambucus nigra with Antimicrobial Activity against Aquaculture Pathogens," *Molecules* 23, no. 5 (May 2018): 1033.

and elderflowers to address numerous health issues, from fighting off viruses to quelling inflammation and supporting circulatory health. Rosemary Gladstar contends that "elder flowers and berries are some of the best medicine and food we have" and praises their effectiveness in treating viral infections and fever.[40] Herbalist jim mcdonald has called elder "among the most revered of herbs."[41]

I had the pleasure of speaking at length about elder to Rosalee de la Forêt, a registered herbalist and author of *Alchemy of Herbs: Transform Everyday Ingredients into Foods and Remedies that Heal*. I'm a fan of hers because she skillfully brings together the science of nutrition and medical research with her training in herbalism and Chinese medicine. She told me elder is "one of my very favorite plants . . . one I rely on all the time."

One of the central tenets of her book and her practice is that herbalism should treat the person rather than the illness. So while elderberry may be used broadly by most people for preventing cold and flu, having an understanding of an individual's constitution can make it far more effective for supporting overall health, not just in acute situations.

De la Forêt's book goes into some detail about the ways herbalists think about a plant's action in the body. She explains that understanding "energetics," which refers both to the ways plants tend to make us feel and to the typical states of our own bodies, can help us tailor the use of herbs like elder to our particular needs. Herbalists typically classify energetics into four categories—hot, cold, dry, and damp—which can apply to a person, plant, or illness. Considering energetics can make herbal remedies more targeted, for instance if you're trying to treat a dry cough rather than a wet, phlegmy one, or if you tend to feel cold or hot. Different parts of plants collected at different times in the growing season and prepared in different ways may also vary in their effects.

She notes that elderberry is "cooling, but not dramatically so." If you tend to run cold, de la Forêt says, the cooling effect of elderberry can be counteracted by adding warming spices like ginger, black pepper, or rosemary to your preparations. She recommends taking small doses throughout the day when you're dealing with a cold or fever, and she sometimes takes a spoonful twice per hour if she feels she's fighting off a virus.

---

40 Rosemary Gladstar, *Medicinal Herbs: A Beginner's Guide* (North Adams, MA: Storey), 134.

41 jim mcdonald, "Elder." herbcraft.org/elder.html

She finds elder useful in less acute situations as well. In *Alchemy of Herbs* she suggests that "herbs and spices will have the most dramatic and positive influence on your health if you maximize their use in your everyday life."[42] She turns to elderberry, "one of our highest antioxidant berries that we use in herbal medicine," to help people address chronic inflammation, adding phytochemicals to diets often lacking in these disease-preventing compounds. She suggests its daily use for heart health and notes that "it's famous for protecting eyes, which are very sensitive to chronic inflammation."

She suggests drinking tea regularly as one of the easiest ways to get frequent doses of this valuable anti-inflammatory herb and often makes a strong unsweetened decoction she drinks warm. She also likes to add elderflowers to baked oatmeal and other baked goods and enjoys mulled elderberry wine. For a deliciously decadent way to enjoy your elderberry, try her recipe for Chocolate Syrup with Elderberry and Rose Hips on page 132.

Because we're all constituted differently, there's no one-size-fits-all approach for using elderberry, or any other herb for that matter. "I recommend that people start with small amounts of herbs, then slowly increase the amount over time," de la Forêt says, in order to "find your own optimal therapeutic dose."[43] She notes that some people are more sensitive to elderberry seeds and will get an upset stomach if they are not strained out of food preparations, as in jam or pie.

Herbalist Lise Wolff recommends very small amounts of elderberry for immune support, just 1 to 3 drops of tincture daily as a preventative "to stimulate the immune system" during cold season. In her practice, she emphasizes herbs as gentle suggestions to the body to heal itself, and uses elderberry tincture at much lower doses than are often recommended, with good results—perhaps too good. She cautions that we should give the body a break from any herb so it can function unsupported. With elderberry, she told me, "I worry it's too effective, and I think it's important that the immune system gets an opportunity to work and go through the fever process and learn how to respond to its environment of its own accord rather than always being assisted." She likens the immune system to a muscle that needs exercise to stay strong, and suggests viewing the occasional cold as an opportunity to let the immune system get practice doing its own fighting rather than using herbs against all viruses.

---

42 Rosalee de la Forêt, *Alchemy of Herbs: Transform Everyday Ingredients into Foods and Remedies that Heal* (Carlsbad, CA: Hay House, 2017), xix.

43 de la Forêt, 29.

Elderflowers have been a staple of herbal medicine for centuries and remain a go-to with contemporary herbalists for treating fevers. Elderflower, de la Forêt says, is "one of my very favorite herbs when somebody has a fever and feels hot, restless, tense," because rather than lowering fever as over-the-counter medications do, elderflower works by promoting sweating to let heat escape, what herbalists call "opening the periphery." This "diaphoretic" or "sudorific" action helps make someone more comfortable while allowing the fever process to counter the infection. De la Forêt points out that the modern impulse to lower all fevers can be counterproductive, as fever is one way our bodies mount an immune response. Elderflower will not immediately reduce fever but, as jim mcdonald explains,

> is a relaxant diaphoretic; which is to say that it encourages perspiration and the release of heat by relaxing tension and resistance in the periphery of the body. It also helps mildly to expectorate phlegm from the lungs & breathways, and so are indicated in fevers accompanied by stuffy sinus or lung congestion. Elderflowers are ever-so-slightly sedative, and help to instill a bit of "ease" that makes getting through a fever a bit more bearable.[44]

Maud Grieve, early twentieth century herbal researcher, notes the traditional use of elderflower infusion to aid recovery, explaining that after giving elderflower tea to someone with a fever, "Heavy perspiration and refreshing sleep will follow, and the patient will wake up well on the way to recovery and the cold or influenza will probably be banished within thirty-six hours."

Wolff also uses elderflower regularly. She's found it helpful for stopping cycles of chronic fever in children and reports that doses of 1 to 3 drops of fresh elderflower tincture have been "remarkably effective" in helping numerous clients resolve pain from endometrial issues. Herbalist Julie Bruton-Seal recommends a cold infusion of elderflower to help with night sweats and menopausal hot flashes or as a diuretic. She also suggests elderflower steeped in glycerine (called a glycerite, more on this below) for sore throats, stuffy noses, and hot flashes, or used as a face lotion.[45]

---

44 mcdonald, "Elder." herbcraft.org/elder.html
45 Julie Bruton-Seal and Matthew Seal, *Backyard Medicine: Harvest and Make Your Own Herbal Remedies* (New York: Castle Books, 2012), 59.

Though many traditional remedies used the elder's leaves, bark, and roots, most herbalists practicing today find their action too extreme. If you do want to experiment with abundant elder leaves, try the soothing balm developed by Jan Berry (a.k.a. The Nerdy Farm Wife) that extracts some of the leaves' healing properties in an infused oil on page 178. Bruton-Seal indicates elder leaf salve for bruises, sprains, and chilblains.

Cautions

As with any herb or supplement, you should pay attention to how you respond to elder and consume in moderation. Herbalist David Winston recommends beginning with only ¼ of the recommended dose the first time you use an herb to ensure you don't have a reaction. He suggests increasing the dose slowly over a two-week period. He also advises heeding dosage guidelines, as many people mistakenly think that if a little is good, more must be better.[46]

Remember when using herbs with children that their smaller bodies need proportionately less herb. Though elderberry and elderflower are generally considered safe for kids, a fifty-pound child should probably get no more than a third of any recommended dosages, which are generally targeted at 150-pound adults. If you're including additional herbs in your preparations, consult one of the books in the resources section to make sure those herbs are considered safe for children, as not all are.

You should speak with your doctor before consuming elderberry or elderflower if you have a chronic medical condition or take certain medications, like immunosuppressants, corticosteroids, medications for diabetes, or Theophylline, a respiratory medication used for asthma and COPD. If you are undergoing chemotherapy or take diuretics or laxatives, elderberry may not be recommended. Winston notes that some herbs may decrease or increase the absorption of medications or may enhance or decrease the activity of certain drugs. A small number of people may have an allergic reaction after consuming elderberry or elderflower.

---

46 David Winston, "Herbal Usage Guidelines." davidwinston.org/dw-guidance.html

Have you heard elderberry plants called "toxic" or "poisonous"? There's a fair amount of dispute about the veracity of these statements. It's important to understand that people use these terms in different, and not always technically accurate, ways. Though some "poisons" and other "toxic" substances are deadly, some will only make you feel sick. The stems and seeds of elderberry are often labeled "mildly toxic," which, as you might imagine, doesn't mean they will kill you. How much one consumes also factors in, and more than one researcher I spoke to pointed out that even something as innocuous—even vital to life—as water can kill you if you drink too much. Now, elder plants do contain compounds that can make you very ill, especially if consumed in large amounts or if you're one of the people very sensitive to them. Remember elder leaves, bark, and roots were used as emetics, that is, they will cause vomiting, so it's generally recommended to consume only the flowers and ripe berries.

Most parts of the European (*S. nigra*) elderberry plant, including the berries and flowers, contain varying amounts of alkaloids and other substances that may cause nausea, as well as common plant compounds called cyanogenic glycosides, which can release cyanide when broken down. (Yes, like the poison murderers in detective novels use, that cyanide. Not what you want in a "health food!") Many food plants contain them, some in large amounts, like cassava and bamboo shoots, requiring special processing to make them safe to eat. Other foods you likely enjoy on a regular basis contain smaller amounts, including almonds, lima beans, chickpeas, and many others we eat without concern of poisoning.

I spent untold hours searching for a definitive answer to how concerned we should be about the cyanogenic glycosides in elderberries. One book I consulted called the warnings about them "phytohysteria," while a researcher I spoke with labeled many of the warnings about cyanide in elderberries on the internet "hogwash." There are several reasons we may have less to worry about than the folks calling elderberry "poisonous" would lead us to believe, though considering the confusion about these compounds, their caution is certainly understandable. First, these compounds are far more concentrated in leaves and stems (which we don't eat) than in the ripe berries and flowers.[47] Second, research conducted at the University of Missouri on midwestern *canadensis* plants found that the native elderberries they analyzed contained negligible amounts of cyanogenic

---

47   Denis Charlebois et al., "Elderberry: Botany, Horticulture, Potential." *Horticultural Reviews* 37 (2010).

glycosides.[48] Concentrations are generally higher in *nigra* varieties, but according to University of Leeds food biochemistry professor Michael Morgan "the levels of cyanogenic glycosides in elderberries is VERY low."

Aside from the concern about cyanide, other components in uncooked elderberries may be involved in the gastrointestinal problems some people have reported after consuming them. One possible culprit is lectin, the compound in many beans that can make people violently ill if they consume insufficiently cooked legumes.[49] Some people may be especially sensitive to lectins or have allergies to a particular protein in elderberries, but cooking helps to deactivate them. A 2017 experiment found that "short-time heat treatment reduces potential allergy-related risks deriving from elderberry consumption without seriously affecting its properties as an antioxidant," and the USDA affirms that cooked elderberries are safe to consume.[50] The one documented case of poisoning (i.e., sickening, not fatal) from elderberry occurred when fresh *S. mexicana* leaves and branches were pressed with the berries and consumed in large quantities as uncooked juice. Several people who drank the juice got very ill and were treated at a nearby hospital. All affected recovered.[51] (A number of people have, however, died from consuming too much water.)[52]

---

48 Andrew Thomas, personal communication. His presentation on the subject can be found here: great-plainsgrowersconference.org/uploads/2/9/1/4/29140369/elderberry_cyanide_st._joe_january_2019.pdf A 1998 study of wild *canadensis* plants found negligible amounts in most leaf material analyzed. R. A. Buhrmester et. al, "Sambunigrin and Cyanogenic Variability in Populations of *Sambucus canadensis L.* (Caprifoliaceae)." *Biochemical Systematics and Ecology* 28, no. 7 (August 1, 2000): 689–695.

49 Laurie C. Dolan et al., "Naturally Occurring Food Toxins," *Toxins* (Basel) 2, no. 9 (September 2010): 2289–2332.

50 Pilar Jiménes et al., "Lectin Digestibility and Stability of Elderberry Antioxidants to Heat Treatment In Vitro." *Molecules* 22, no.1 (January 201): 95.
     United States Department of Agriculture, "Common Elderberry." plants.usda.gov/plantguide/pdf/cs_sanic4.pdf

51 Centers for Disease Control and Prevention, "Poisoning from Elderberry Juice—California" *Morbidity and Mortality Weekly Report* 33. No. 13 (April 06, 1984): 173–4. cdc.gov/mmwr/preview/mmwrhtml/00000311.htm This notice mentions "older, anecdotal reports of poisoning in children from the related elder, *S. canadensis*," but I can find no record of them. Foraging expert Steve Brill urges caution using the wood, reporting that "Children have been poisoned using elderberry-twig peashooters, and adults have been poisoned using hollow twigs to tap maple trees." [Steve Brill, *Identifying and Harvesting Edible and Medicinal Plants in Wild (and Not So Wild) Places* (New York: Harper Collins, 1994), 105.] Since elder wood has long been used for these purposes, I wonder if the wood used was fresh and green, and therefore more liable to leach juice containing the substances of concern. Best to be cautious if you make things from elder branches that might have contact with food or go in your mouth!

52 Coco Ballantyne, "Strange but True: Drinking Too Much Water Can Kill." *Scientific American* (June 21, 2007). "Drinking too Much Water Can be Fatal to Athletes." *Science Daily* (September 2, 2014).

In my efforts to understand the intricacies of elderberry's reported toxicity, I talked to Dennis Lubahn, Director of the University of Missouri's Center on Botanical Interactions Studies, who oversaw a number of recent federally-funded studies looking at elderberry's effect on several health conditions. His answer to my questions about rendering cyanogenic glycosides safe: "Nobody knows." He explained that the way modern scientific inquiry works means that the expensive studies we might need to definitively answer such questions aren't always practical. However, he told me, "There's a lot of really cool stuff that humanity has figured out over the last ten thousand years by trial and error, by people walking through the forest sampling leaves and seeing what happened." Likewise, the traditions handed down over centuries involving cooking the berries for a period of time indicate that trials and errors had proven it a best practice. "That's what people have been doing for hundreds of years," he explained. "It works," even if we don't know exactly why. I found this perspective from a professional biochemist very reassuring, and for now, it's the best information we've got.

The upshot of all this inquiry:

1. Eating raw berries or too many seeds may give some more sensitive people gastrointestinal distress, but cooked berries and things made from them in moderate amounts are considered safe and are well tolerated by most people.
2. Berries from *canadensis* varieties likely contain smaller amounts of cyanogenic glycosides than *nigra* varieties, and both may contain less than you get from other foods you eat regularly.
3. Consuming leaves, stems, bark, or roots of some elderberry plants may send you to the hospital—so please don't! Stick to the berries and flowers.

Pregnant women and babies: elderberries have not been studied for safety in pregnancy or for babies, so it's currently recommended to avoid them.

Those with autoimmune conditions: Elderberry's ability to stimulate the immune system has led to some concern that it may worsen autoimmune conditions.

A systematic review conducted in 2014 also recommended caution with elderberry due to concerns over ingesting cyanogenic glucosides for people with arrhythmias or cardiovascular disease, CNS disorders, dermatological conditions, gastrointestinal disorders, or those taking blood pressure medications.

Now that you've paid careful attention to the cautions and potential hazards of elderberry, let's look at the ways we can use it to support health.

Supporting Immune Function with Elderberry

While elderberry may benefit your health in multiple ways, most people seek it out to keep winter colds and flu to a minimum. Here's what to know about using elderberries to defend yourself from the germs going around during cold season.

UNDERSTANDING IMMUNE SUPPORT

While elderberry has developed something of a reputation as an "immune booster," it's important to understand that the immune system is a very complex thing, involving numerous different bodily processes. While elderberry seems to have an impressive ability to interfere with viral replication, taking regular doses of elderberry doesn't guarantee you'll never catch another cold, especially if you don't do other things to support immune function. Let's take a closer look at what's involved in keeping the immune system working effectively.

A lot of us live overly busy, high-stress lives and short ourselves on sleep, exercise, and time outdoors. You probably know intuitively that when you're exhausted or stressed, you're more likely to get sick, which research supports.[53] Your body needs adequate rest to repair itself. The cortisol your body pumps out when you're under stress over the long term also makes it harder for the components of your immune system to function. One simple way to reduce cortisol and sleep better: Spend time outdoors, as research suggests that contact with nature can reduce stress, while natural sunlight helps regulate our sleep cycles.[54] The exercise we get when we go for a stroll helps, too!

53 Agnese Mariotti, "The Effects of Chronic Stress on Health: New Insights into the Molecular Mechanisms of Brain–Body Communication," *Future Science OA* 1, no. 3 (November 2015): FSO23.
    Jennifer N. Morey et al., "Current Directions in Stress and Human Immune Function," *Current Opinion in Psychology* 5 (October 2015): 13–17.
    Luciana Besedovsky et al., "Sleep and Immune Function," *Pflugers Archive* 463, no. 1 (January 2012): 121–137.
54 Nathaniel P. Morris, "Take Two Hikes and Call Me in the Morning," *Scientific American* (September 17, 2017). blogs.scientificamerican.com/observations/take-2-hikes-and-call-me-in-the-morning/

Cover all your bases by taking a good long walk foraging elderflowers, elderberries, and other wild foods. Contact with nature, downtime, exercise, sun, plus yummy medicinal ingredients for your home apothecary—a multitasking move for better health if I ever heard one.

Another key issue to keep in mind is the role of our diet in maintaining or sabotaging health. Our immune systems require many different nutrients to function well, and the Standard American Diet (known by the fitting acronym SAD) falls short on a lot of them. If you're eating a diet of mostly processed foods that include a lot of refined flour, sugar, and oil, you're likely missing out on some nutrients your immune system needs. Yes, vitamin C is one of them, but it turns out there are lots more vitamins and minerals involved, and a deficiency in just one may set you up for more frequent viral infections, from colds to flu. Some of the most critical players:

- Vitamin A
- B-6
- B-12
- Folate
- Vitamin C
- Vitamin D
- Vitamin E
- Magnesium
- Copper
- Selenium
- Zinc

If you don't tend to eat many vegetables and fruits, you're probably missing some of these nutrients. Conversely, if you eat mainly a vegetarian or vegan diet, a number of these nutrients can be hard to source from plants. You need to be mindful and make sure you're getting the recommended daily allowances of things like iron, B-6, and B-12, which are more readily available in animal products.

Nutrition experts advise that getting nutrients from foods rather than supplements is generally preferable, as isolated vitamins and minerals don't always work the same way in our bodies as those derived from whole foods. Additionally, some supplements may contain doses far larger than you need and can do more harm than good, so use them sparingly and with caution, and seek the advice of your doctor. Working in more whole foods high in the nutrients you lack may help your immune system function more effectively.

Because research into the human microbiome—those trillions of bacteria that live in our digestive tracts—continues to demonstrate the vital role of the gut in immune function, supporting it with your food choices provides another line of defense against common illnesses. For that reason, the recipes here mostly avoid sugar and refined ingredients, which research suggests disrupts the balance of gut flora.[55] To keep your gut working well, focus on a whole-foods diet rich in fibrous plants, and incorporate fermented foods like yogurt, kefir, and lacto-fermented vegetables. The fermented elderberry recipes here count! Try some Elderberry Kombucha (page 161), homemade Sun-Extracted Elderberry Wine (page 166), or Fermented Elderberry and Honey Soda (page 152).[56]

Even if you eat a balanced whole-foods diet, get enough rest, wash your hands often, and keep stress under control, sometimes viruses still find a way to get a foothold. Having some elderberry and elderflower preparations at the ready may help you fight back and evade a cold or shorten its duration.

Will taking elderberry mean you'll never get sick again? Probably not. But you may find yourself among the few people who stay healthy when everyone around them has taken ill. Some devotees take their favorite elderberry preparation hourly when they feel something coming on and find they never actually come down with anything. Or perhaps your bout of flu will be mercifully short and mild, as the people in the Israeli and Norwegian studies found. Regardless, those potent antioxidants will do your body good in other ways even if you do succumb to the occasional cold.

GETTING THE MOST OUT OF YOUR ELDERBERRIES

Preparations that extract the most beneficial compounds from elderberries generally rely on heat or time. The most potent preparations will require simmering, steeping in water, or tincturing in a solvent.

---

55 M. K. Zinöcker and I. A. Lindseth, "The Western Diet-Microbiome-Host Interaction and Its Role in Metabolic Disease," *Nutrients* 10, no. 3 (Mar 17, 2018): pii: E365.
    W. Kruis et al., "Effect of Diets Low and High in Refined Sugars on Gut Transit, Bile Acid Metabolism, and Bacterial Fermentation," 32, no. 4 (April 1991): 367–371.

56 Emerging research also suggests that exposure to chemically-based household disinfectants can disrupt our microbiomes, so while you're pursuing these wonderful natural remedies, do yourself a favor and make sure your cleaning routine depends on the power of plants, too. Mon H. Tun et al., "Postnatal Exposure to Household Disinfectants, Infant Gut Microbiota and Subsequent Risk of Overweight in Children" *CMAJ* 190, no. 37 (September 17, 2018): E1097–E1107.

When you're brewing tea for medicinal purposes, the quick dunk you might give your usual tea bag just isn't enough time to extract the medicinal compounds we're after. For infusions of elderflower, plan to steep for no less than ten minutes, but ideally allow it to infuse four to ten hours before straining.[57]

Dried berries, which are a little tougher and less ready to infuse into hot water, need a good simmer to extract their medicinal compounds and reduce levels of cyanogenic glycosides in dried berries. Twenty to thirty minutes over low heat is the standard recommendation, and as I mention in the recipe section, a second or even third simmer with fresh water will continue to yield a dark, reasonably flavorful tea. You'll definitely be able to taste for yourself that much of the berries' flavor transferred to your first batch. Though likely less powerful medicinally, this second brewing tastes good and probably contains at least some of elderberry's beneficial compounds.

For longer-lasting remedies you can keep in your pantry, you need to add alcohol or a great deal of sugar to prevent spoilage. You can extend the shelf life of homemade elderberry syrup by adding alcohol or extra sweetener, as explained in the recipe section.

Another option is tincturing, which means soaking something in high-proof alcohol for four to eight weeks. A tincture extracts plant compounds slowly over time, and different ones than those extracted by water. One big advantage of tinctures is that since they're preserved in alcohol, they keep for years, rather than the few months of syrups made without alcohol. However, given how often it's recommended we take elderberry for fighting viruses, de la Forêt points out, using the typically recommended amounts (4–6 ml) of elderberry tincture every hour would mean consuming quite a bit of alcohol, so tincture isn't her first choice for using elder in acute situations.

Lise Wolff's clients have had success using her low-dosage technique of just 1 to 3 drops twice per day if they've been exposed to something, and up to ten drops 3 to 4 times per day if they're coming down with something. If you prefer to avoid alcohol, you can use glycerine instead (making what's called a glycerite), but most herbalists say glycerine isn't as effective at extracting herbal compounds as alcohol.

You can also make an oxymel, a mixture involving roughly one part berries, one part apple cider vinegar, and one part honey (page 111).

---

57 Maria Noël Groves, *Body into Balance: An Herbal Guide to Holistic Self-Care* (North Adams, MA: Storey, 2016), 302, and "Long Herbal Infusions" wildwoodinstitute.com/articles/long-herbal-infusions.html

HERBAL TERMS TO KNOW

Tea—A small amount of herb steeped for a short time in boiling water, though some herbalists use the word tea to describe a small amount of decoction diluted in water.

Infusion—A larger amount of herb, usually 1 to 3 tablespoons per cup, steeped in boiling water for a longer amount of time (often several hours) to extract more of the compounds from the herb. Infusions are generally used for the leaves and flowers of plants.

Decoction—The tougher parts of plants, like berries, roots, and bark, require simmering in hot water to extract the compounds from the plant.

Tincture—A tincture typically uses alcohol to extract compounds from the plant over the course of several weeks. Very small amounts are used medicinally. Vinegar may also be used to make what's technically called an acetum.

Glycerite—Uses glycerine instead of alcohol to extract herbal compounds.

Oxymel—Herbs steeped in a combination of vinegar and honey for several weeks.

Using Elderberries for Immune Support

Most of us turn to elderberry preparations when we feel we're coming down with something, but many elderberry fans take a preventative daily spoonful of elderberry syrup throughout cold and flu season. A daily cup of elderberry tea or a small dose of tincture would be other options, though there's some disagreement about the usefulness or potential downsides of taking elderberry every day. Whether or not you're fighting off illness, the antioxidants in both elderberry and elderflower have a wide range of benefits, especially for helping counter the chronic inflammation so many of us have as a result of stress, exposure to chemicals, and poor diet.

When you know there's something going around or someone in
your family feels a little under the
weather, dosing frequently with
elderberry may help your immune
system fight off infection before it
can take hold. If they do come down
with something, the illness may be
milder and quicker than without
elderberry. As we've learned from the
in vitro studies, elderberry appears
to stimulate the immune response,
while also blocking viruses' ability to
penetrate cells in the early stages of
illness and interfering with replication in the later stages, which helps
to explain why people recover more
quickly with elderberry than without.

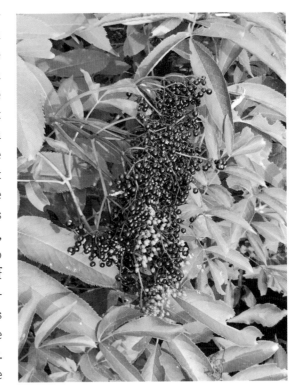

De la Forêt explained to me
there is no definitive guide to dos-
ing with elderberry. The amounts typically used in Ayurveda and Chinese medicine, she says, are much greater than in western herbalism, and some western
herbalists use far less or more than others. You may want to start with the very
low doses Wolff suggests and use more if you feel it's not helping.

De la Forêt favors a strong unsweetened decoction made with one cup
(115 grams) of dried elderberries simmered in one cup of water and recommends
taking this preparation frequently in the early stages of illness, one teaspoon to
one tablespoon every hour. I find an unsweetened decoction preferable as well,
as a spoonful of syrup every hour is a lot of added sugar. You can take decoction
plain by the spoonful or dilute it in hot water as a tea. When she travels, de la
Forêt always brings a tincture of elderberry and echinacea, taking four to six ml
up to eight times per day to fend off the viruses we're exposed to on planes.

For elderberry syrups, she likes to add rose hips, which contain natural pec-
tin to thicken the syrup. She includes licorice, thyme, and rosemary in her homemade syrup, and suggests a spoonful every hour, or even every half hour, at the
first sign of a cold.

Elderberry gummies are a fun way to get a dose of elderberry and other herbs if we include them. The gelatin they're made with is also rich in protein, helpful for getting in some nutrition when appetites are blunted by infection. Some natural health experts believe gelatin also supports gut health, which in turn may make our immune systems function more effectively.

Tea is a great choice for keeping bodies hydrated during illness, and adding honey can help with sore throats and coughs. Popsicles made from elderberry tea or elderberry cut with juice are another option for hydrating and soothing sore throats. Choose a juice with some vitamin C in it for additional immune support. Drops and lollipops (see recipes on pages 115 and 116) are another way to get tasty doses of elderberry while helping to control coughs and soothe irritated throat tissue.

ADDITIONAL INGREDIENTS TO CONSIDER

These elderberry preparations work well on their own, but we can also add any number of immune-supporting herbs for additional benefits. You can expand the uses for your elderberry preparations by making syrups, teas, and tinctures that include complementary herbs for things like immune support, allergy relief, or cough suppression.

Be sure to do your homework. Consult one of the herbal handbooks or websites in the resources section to check for contraindications. While many ingredients below are common kitchen spices, some herbs are not recommended during pregnancy, for nursing mothers, or for children under two years old. Heed the guidelines mentioned in the caution section about trying new herbs slowly and consult your doctor about possible drug interactions or concerns with existing health conditions.

Also bear in mind de la Forêt's advice to consider the energetics of the herb and its effect on you. Just because a given herb works well for your friend doesn't mean it will act the same way in your body.

This is not an exhaustive list of possible additions, but rather some options to get you started incorporating other herbal remedies.

FOR FIGHTING OFF VIRUSES

Astragalus root

A popular herbal medicine for immune support, de la Forêt touts astragalus as "a supreme herb for the immune system," and research has explored its effects.[58] She recommends including 10 to 30 grams per day over a long period of time for sustained protection against colds (as well as additional benefits like increased energy). The root may be simmered with your elderberries for use in tea, syrups, or other recipes calling for a decoction of berries.

Echinacea

Echinacea has long been a go-to herb for its antibacterial and antiviral properties. The mainstream news media has gotten people pretty confused about echinacea, in large part because the studies on its effectiveness against colds have used different varieties of plant, different parts of the plant, and varying preparations (teas, tinctures, pills).[59] Rosemary Gladstar writes that "Many herbalists and natural-medicine practitioners feel it's the most important immune-enhancing herb in Western medicine." She advises, "Echinacea is always more effective if taken at the early signs of illness, before the illness has the opportunity to 'settle in.' Echinacea is particularly effective against bronchial and respiratory infections, and in any situation where the immune system needs fortifying."[60] Most herbalists don't recommend taking it regularly, only when you feel like you might be coming down with something or have been exposed.

If you grow echinacea, Gladstar suggests making a whole-plant tincture, steeped over the course of the growing season, including new leaves in late spring, buds, then flowers, then roots at the end of season. A tincture made from the fresh, rather than dried, root is considered most effective if you have access to plants. You may also make a tincture of dried echinacea root or add roots and flowers to decoctions targeting the early stage of illness.

---

58 De la Forêt, 308; Juan Fu et. al, "Review of the Botanical Characteristics, Phytochemistry, and Pharmacology of *Astragalus membranaceus* (Huangqi) *Phytotherapy Research* 28, no. 9 (September 2014): 1275–1283.

59 Stephanie M. Ross, "Echinacea Purpurea: A Proprietary Extract of Echinacea Purpurea is Shown to be Safe and Effective in the Prevention of the Common Cold." *Holistic Nurse Practitioner* 30, no. 1 (Jan-Feb 2016): 54–7.
   Sachin A. Shah et al., "Evaluation of Echinacea for the Prevention and Treatment of the Common Cold: A Meta-Analysis." *The Lancet Infectious Diseases* 7, no. 1 (July 1, 2007): 473–480. thelancet.com /journals/laninf/article/PIIS1473-3099%2807%2970160–3/fulltext

60 Gladstar, 129–30.

Rose Hips

A rich source of vitamin C when picked fresh, rose hips are a common addition to elderberry syrup recipes, though their vitamin C is greatly reduced by drying and cooking. In *The New Healing Herbs*, Michael Castleman reports that "the drying process destroys 45 to 90 percent of it, and infusions extract only about 40 percent of what's left."[61]

If you don't have fresh rose hips on hand, dried ones have benefits apart from vitamin C. Like elderberries, rose hips contain antioxidants, and in clinical trials their anti-inflammatory abilities have helped alleviate arthritis pain, while *in vitro* and animal experiments suggest their usefulness for inflammatory conditions like diabetes and obesity, as well as kidney, liver, and neurological disease. They also have antimicrobial properties.[62]

Ginger

Both fresh and dried ginger may serve numerous purposes, soothing sore throats and body aches, quelling inflammation, and relieving congestion. Ginger may also work as an antiviral, especially in fresh form.[63] De la Forêt advises, "If you could choose only one herb to use during a cold or the flu, ginger might be the one, especially when there are signs of coldness and dampness such as shivering or a thickly coated tongue."[64] She recommends using fresh rather than dried ginger for colds but suggests avoiding it if someone already feels overheated and dry.

Black Pepper

It can seem a little odd to put black pepper in something sweet like an elderberry syrup, but de la Forêt recommends it as "a wonderful activator herb that helps other herbs be more effective."[65] Studies looking at the bioavailability of turmeric found that adding the active compound in black pepper, piperine, increases bioavailability up to 2000 percent.

---

61 Michael Castleman *The New Healing Herbs*, (New York: Rodale: 2009), 402.

62 Inés Mármol et al., "Therapeutic Applications of Rose Hips from Different Rosa Species." *International Journal of Molecular Science* 18, no. 6 (June 2017): 1137.

63 J. S. Chang et al., "Fresh ginger (Zingiber officinale) has Anti-Viral Activity Against Human Respiratory Syncytial Virus in Human Respiratory Tract Cell Lines." *Journal of Ethnopharmacology* 145, no. 1 (Jan 9, 2013): 1 46–51.

64 de la Forêt, 90.

65 de la Forêt, "Elderberry Gummy Recipe," learningherbs.com/remedies-recipes/gummy-bear-recipe/

Cloves

Besides being delicious, cloves are antimicrobial and anti-inflammatory, soothing on sore throats, and work as an expectorant. They also aid digestion.

Cinnamon

Rosemary Gladstar recommends cinnamon as "a powerful antiseptic, with antiviral and antifungal properties . . . often indicated in cases of viral infections."[66] Cinnamon is often used for fevers and coughs, and as a warming spice that makes things taste good. Cassia and ceylon cinnamon are used similarly by herbalists, but the stronger-flavored cassia cinnamon should be consumed in moderation because of possible harmful effects from too much of the coumarin it contains.[67]

Calendula

De la Forêt calls calendula "a premier herb for the skin and mucus membranes." She also says it "relieves inflammation, increases beneficial immune responses, is mildly antimicrobial."[68] Herbalist Jessica Godino counsels, "Calendula gently supports the immune system, especially during times of transition . . . by stimulating lymphatic drainage. The lymph is an essential part of the immune system, filtering and eliminating waste products and bacteria as well as producing infection-fighting cells. Calendula is also anti-microbial and anti-viral."[69]

Licorice Root

A staple in traditional Chinese medicine, licorice root is used in small amounts in combination with other herbs for its soothing and antiviral properties.[70] It has a slippery feel ("demulcent" in herbal speak) that makes it a natural for soothing sore throats and coughs, as well as supporting gut health. Licorice is not recommended in large amounts or for extended periods of time, as it can raise blood pressure and reduce potassium levels.

---

66 Gladstar, 65.

67 K. Abraham et al., "Toxicology and Risk Assessment of Coumarin: Focus on Human Data." *Molecular Nutrition and Food Research* 54, no.2 (February 2010): 228–39.

68 De la Forêt, "Calendula Benefits." herbalremediesadvice.org/calendula-benefits.html

69 Jessica Godino. "Calendula." susunweed.com/An_Article_wisewoman3c.htm

70 Liqiang Wang, "The Antiviral and Antimicrobial Activities of Licorice, a Widely-Used Chinese Herb," *Acta Pharmaceutica Sinica* B 5, no. 4 (July 2015): 310–315.

FOR COUGHS AND SORE THROATS

You can add other herbs to infusions, decoctions, or syrups to help control a cough or soothe a sore throat. Some popular options for coughs include hyssop, horehound, thyme, lemon balm, slippery elm, linden, wild cherry bark, cinnamon, mullein, and elecampane. You can also easily forage some cough-soothing ingredients like violet leaves, plantain, and pine needles.

Sore throats may benefit from sage, licorice, marshmallow, or mullein, which you could add to syrups or decoctions that can be turned into tea, popsicles, or throat lozenges.

FOR FEVERS

A traditional combination for addressing fevers is a combination of equal parts elderflower, yarrow, and peppermint, which Gladstar calls "Gypsy Cold Care." Both yarrow and elderflower are used to induce sweating and lower fever. She recommends the combination for seasonal allergies and sinus congestion as well. You can make the tea yourself or buy it ready-made from the company Gladstar founded, Traditional Medicinals. It's widely available in grocery stores and online. Elderflower and yarrow may also be added to bath water to alleviate fever as well.

FOR SEASONAL ALLERGIES

Elderflower is often used to help with hayfever, and it may be combined with additional herbs that tame seasonal allergies in infusions you drink before allergy season begins. Nettle and goldenrod are thought especially effective for this purpose, and astragalus may help as well. Elderberry's antioxidants, especially quercitin, may also help alleviate allergy symptoms.

FOR CALMING INFLAMMATION

Elderberry can be combined with other powerful anti-inflammatory herbs and spices, notably ginger, turmeric, nettle, and rose hips.

FOR EXTERNAL USE

Both the flowers and leaves of the elder are used for treating sprains, bruises, and skin irritation, usually in infused oils and salves. Combine elderflower with calendula and chamomile in a soothing skin balm or make a poultice with the flower or leaves combined with common yard "weeds" plantain and yarrow.

Brent Madding, who grows seven thousand elderberry plants primarily for their flowers at 360 Farms in Webbers Falls, Oklahoma, stumbled upon elderflower's skin-nourishing capacities by accident. A hard-working farmer with hands that showed it, after harvesting and processing his elder blossoms, he was stunned to see that his hands had "no cracks, no bleeding, and the calluses were gone." He jokes, "I had the hands of a ninth-floor banker," rather than a farmer. This first-hand experience of elderflower's beneficial impact on skin prompted his wife to develop a line of soaps and moisturizers featuring elderflower.

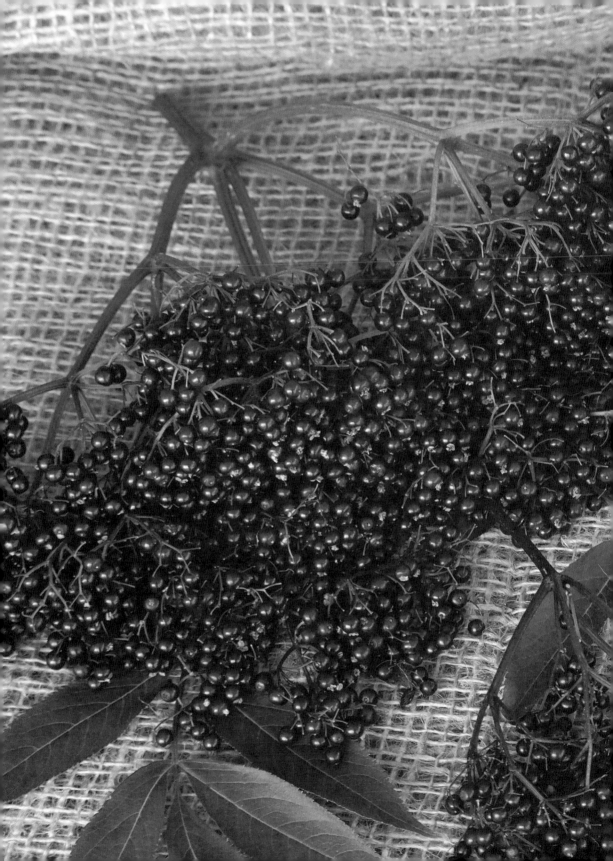

CHAPTER 3

SOURCING ELDERBERRIES AND ELDERFLOWERS

"It has been said, with some truth, that our English summer is not here until the Elder is fully in flower, and that it ends when the berries are ripe."
—Maud Grieve, *A Modern Herbal*, 1931

The most cost effective (and in many people's opinion, fun) way to obtain elderflowers and elderberries is foraging, as they grow wild in most of North America as well as in much of Europe. But foraging isn't for everyone for a variety of reasons. Not all of us have easy access to elderberry shrubs, though you can find elderberries growing even in many metropolitan areas. And of course foraging takes time, which is often in short supply. No worries! You can still easily—even economically—get the benefits of elderberries. If you lack the time, interest, ability, or courage to forage, elderberries and elderberry preparations have become widely available for purchase in stores and online.

What to Look for When Buying Elderberries and Elderflowers

You probably won't find fresh elderberries or elderflowers for sale at your local grocery store, though you may find someone selling them at a farmers' market, and a few local elderberry growers may have elderflowers or fresh, frozen, or juiced berries for sale. A search at localharvest.org can help you locate nearby elderberry farms, whose numbers have been growing in recent years. Most people who want fresh berries and flowers forage them, but as the market for elderberry expands, you may begin seeing more on offer.

What you will find at natural food stores and through online herb sellers are dried berries and flowers. Buy organic when possible, and watch out for stems, leaves, and twigs that sometimes make their way into bags of dried elderberries and elderflowers. I've sometimes found some sizable twigs in my berries, and the package of flowers I bought to compare to the ones I foraged contained far more stem than I had the patience to pick out. Get out as much as you can before using.

You can purchase dried elderberries (mainly *nigra*) by the pound online, or see if your local natural foods store carries them. You can buy them in just the quantity you need in the bulk aisle. Online at major retailers you can find them least expensively by the pound, but they're also sold in smaller quantities. When you find them on sale, they might be as low as $15 per pound, but $20 is pretty average. Plan ahead if you're buying online: Prices can go up significantly in winter, when the fall harvest has mostly sold off and supplies run low.

You can also buy pre-bagged elderberry tea or tea with elderberry extract, but it's far more expensive and not actually much easier than popping some berries in a teacup with a built-in infuser. You'll save a lot of money (and cut the waste of individually-packaged tea) buying the whole berries. It's likely you'll get a more powerful dose of the compounds you're after (and cut down on the cyanogenic ones) if you simmer them on the stove, but if all you're up for is a simple brewed tea, go for it!

Dried elderflowers are a bit pricey, but a little goes a long way. They're available by the pound and in smaller quantities from several companies that specialize in bulk herbs.

There are also numerous pre-made syrups, tinctures, and capsules if you want to try elderberry concoctions without spending time in the kitchen. DIY isn't for everyone, so don't feel bad if that's more your speed. Do whatever works for you. Just a warning: Pre-made elderberry preparations cost far more than making your own. Also, some contain a lot of sugar and preservatives, which may undermine the benefits you're hoping to derive from your berries.

Be mindful of other "immune-boosting" ingredients elderberries may have been combined with. Elderberry and zinc are often paired, but since taking too much zinc can interfere with the absorption of other important minerals it may actually *inhibit* immune function.[1] One popular elderberry lozenge has five milligrams of zinc per candy, while another has twelve, so it's easy to exceed the RDA if you take several over the course of a day. Be sure to read labels so you know what you're getting and don't inadvertently overdo.

---

1   National Institutes of Health, Zinc Professional Fact Sheet. ods.od.nih.gov/factsheets/Zinc-Health Professional/

Foraging Elderberries and Elderflowers

If you're up for a little adventure, foraging elderflowers and elderberries is a delightful way to begin getting to know useful wild plants. Putting up loads of immune-boosting berries just as the school year starts is super-satisfying, as is the knowledge of the money saved on these not-inexpensive little berries. Foraging flowers in late spring or early summer will also save a lot opposed to buying, and playing with edible and medicinal flowers in the kitchen is just plain fun. Drying a few flowerheads in early summer can set you up for some potent cold relief the following winter with very little effort and no expense.

Since elder shrubs and trees can be found all over North America and Europe as well as many other parts of the world, foraging is a possibility open to many of us. The subspecies *canadensis* grows from Nova Scotia all the way to Florida and Texas and as far west as Manitoba. The western variety, blue elderberry (*ssp. cerulea*) grows along the Pacific coast, from British Columbia to

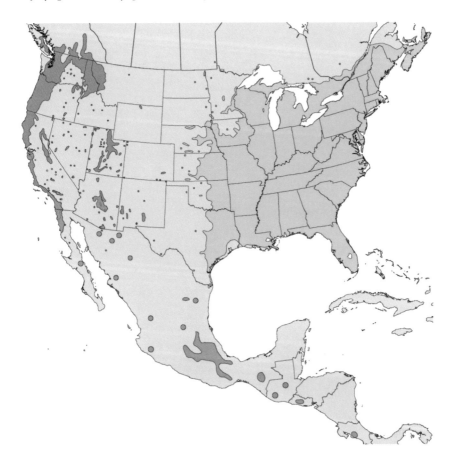

Northern Mexico as far east as Oklahoma. *Sambucus mexicana* grows in desert conditions in Mexico and the American southwest.

Another benefit of foraging (or growing your own), at least if you're in North America, is that you will likely be gathering *canadensis* berries, which may be much lower in cyanogenic compounds than *nigra*. Additionally, access to fresh rather than dried flowers and berries has a number of advantages. Using fresh berries to make juice, syrup, or other preparations likely preserves more of their beneficial compounds if you're careful not to heat them more than necessary (more on this in chapter 5). Also, while dried versions can work for teas, tinctures, and syrup-making, fresh berries and flowers taste better for things like muffins and baked oatmeal, though dried flowers and berries can work. Dried berries can be rehydrated for things like jams and pies, where they will undergo some cooking, and some people say they don't notice much difference between these and fresh berries. But if you intend to extract the ephemeral essence of elderflower for syrups, liqueurs, and all the things you can make with them, picking fresh flowers and using them immediately is the only way to go.

FORAGING BASICS

Know What You're Doing

Whether you're new to foraging or experienced in the practice of wildcrafting, a good field guide is a necessity so you don't inadvertently pick something poisonous! "Wildman" Steve Brill has an info-packed guide called *Identifying & Harvesting Edible and Medicinal Plants*, and Samuel Thayer's *Nature's Garden* is a thorough and highly-regarded foraging book. Going with an experienced forager is an even better way to learn. You can often find classes to get you started getting to know the wild foods in your area.

Remember to use ALL the identifying features of a plant, including leaves, bark, berries, flowers, and siting.

Make sure you're harvesting in areas free from contaminants like herbicides or industrial waste. Roadsides and ditches, and sadly, many public parks are often sprayed with weed killers—not what you want in your health-supporting medicines!

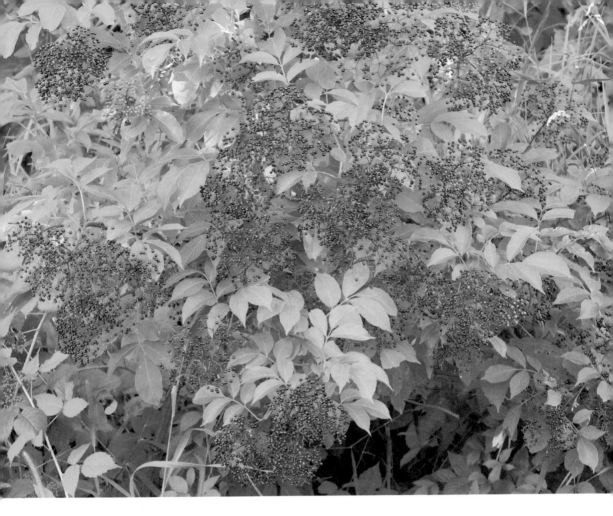

Go Prepared

You'll need a basket, bag, or bucket to collect your flowers and berries. The stems aren't hard to cut, so a simple pair of scissors will suffice unless you're going to collect some wood for crafts, in which case bring along a pair of pruners.

Wear long sleeves and pants to protect from insect bites. Insect-borne diseases are on the rise, and you may head into deer tick territory when you forage elderberries.

Get Permission

If foraging on public land, make sure you check the rules regarding the collection of plant matter. You may need a permit, and there may be limits on what you can take. On private property, make sure to ask permission of the owner.

Harvest Minimally and Respectfully

While it can be exciting to bring home buckets of berries, be sure you're leaving plenty for wildlife and other foragers. Most wildcrafters recommend taking no more than a third of what you find; many suggest taking closer to a tenth. Never take the only one of a flower or plant.

Only take what you will actually use. If you bring home ten gallons of berries but won't have time to process them before they rot, you've wasted time, effort, and food. Be realistic about what you'll be able to do with your harvest.

Also be sure to check whether plants you're foraging are considered endangered or threatened. You can find the listings for your area at the USDA National Resources Conservation Service website by selecting your state.[2] Elderberry is unlikely to be on it, but if you get into foraging other plants, it's important to check.

Try not to disturb other plants or nests on your way to get the berries or flowers you're after.

Identifying Elderberry Shrubs

Novices may be most comfortable connecting with more veteran foragers in their community. You can seek someone through online community groups, or you might find foraging classes offered through nature centers and community education organizations.

If you want to set out foraging on your own, familiarize yourself thoroughly with the distinguishing characteristics of elderberry. Once you've found some elderberry shrubs, you may want to take note of their location to make finding them again easier. Getting to know the flowering and fruiting times in your region will make it more likely you'll catch them at the right times, and also help you avoid their look-alikes. (More on those below.)

Elderberry shrubs tend to grow along streams and the edges of forests and fields, places where their shallow root systems won't be disturbed. In my area, we have a large number growing along train tracks, the edges of farm fields, and on the banks of a nearby stream. Elder is a popular hedgerow plant in England, and London foragers report no difficulty finding plenty of berries and flowers in public ways around the city.

---

2   USDA Natural Resources Conservation Service, "Threatened and Endangered Plants." plants.usda.gov/threat.html

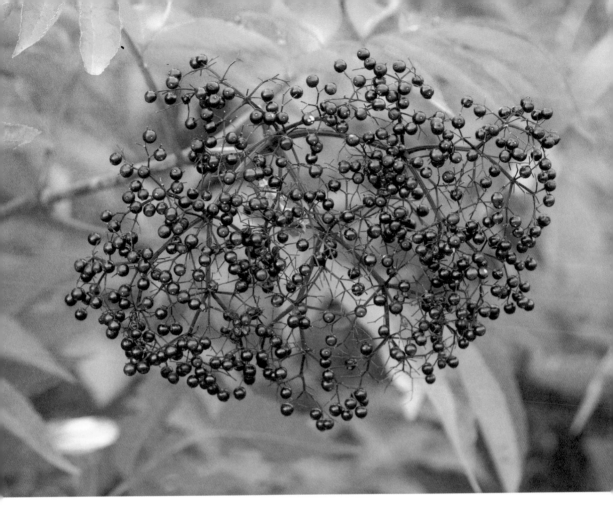

Identification is made easier when the stunning blossoms begin putting on their show as summer begins to heat up. Elderflowers bloom over a several week period in early summer, though timing may be later or earlier depending on the spring weather. The flower heads and berry clusters on a single plant may ripen weeks apart, and plants in shadier locations will bloom later than those in sun, giving foragers plenty of time to gather these lovely blooms and fruits.

You'll find some botanical terms being thrown around when you begin looking at plant identifications. Here's a quick glossary of words that might be unfamiliar:

Pinnate—Leaves are arranged like a feather on opposite sides of an axis.

Compound—Many leaves come off a single stem, in contrast to something like a maple leaf.

Inflorescence—A group or cluster of flowers.

Cyme—A flat cluster of flowers like elderflower, though people often use the word umbel, which describes a cluster of flower stalks.

Herbaceous—Not woody, green and leaf-like.

Lenticels—Raised pores on the bark of the plant that allow gases to penetrate.

Drupe—Technically, elder's berry isn't a berry at all, but a drupe, a fleshy fruit surrounding a seed. You don't actually need to know this to identify elderberry, but you will often see that term applied to it.

IDENTIFYING FEATURES OF ELDERBERRY (AND PLANTS THAT RESEMBLE IT)

→ Remember to use multiple identifying features: leaf arrangement and shape, bark, flower and berry characteristics, and growth habit.

Elderberry shrubs grow from many stems and tend to get six to twelve feet tall, though they can top twenty feet, or even taller in the tree-like growth habit of the western *cerulea*. Their leaves are "pinnately compound," which means an elder leaf is made up of numerous leaflets arranged in a pinnate (like a feather, on opposite sides of an axis), with little or no stalk (petiole) attaching it to the central stem. These long, serrated leaflets with pointed tips grow two to five inches, in groups of five to eleven (typically seven) that can get up to twenty inches in length. They are arranged opposite one another with a terminal leaflet. Bark is light gray and mostly smooth, but with what Thayer describes as "a sparse spackling of warty lenticels."[3] Flowers grow in large flat clusters, which can help distinguish them from plants with similar leaves or berries. Each individual elder blossom is only about ¼-inch in diameter and has five petals and five stamens protruding. When you get to know them you'll realize how easily recognizable they are.

Berries are dark blue, purple, or nearly black when ripe, and hang in large clusters. The *cerulea's* berries are larger and bluer when ripe, and are typically coated with a white dusting of a naturally-occurring yeast.

Different regions will have different subspecies of elder, so get familiar with your local variety as well as other varieties of elder to avoid. In much of North America, the earlier-blooming red elder (*S. racemosa*) is most confused with the sought-after *canadensis*, and in Europe, it's the dwarf elder. Both are described in more detail below. Though both have been used medicinally, the berries and flowers from these plants are more likely to make you ill and are best avoided. Stick with the more edible elderberries: *nigra, canadensis,* and *cerulea.*

Untrained eyes have mistaken other flowers and berries for elders, but using the numerous features of the elderberry plant (not just one) makes correctly identifying them more certain. You should never assume a dark berry or a cluster of flowers is elder unless you've also considered other distinguishing characteristics like its growth habit, leaf pattern, bark, and so on.

Certain shrubs have somewhat similar flowers or fruits, so don't pick a cluster of flowers or berries without checking they're in the right shape (a flat cyme, not a cone shape, for example) on a plant with the right arrangement and type of leaves and bark. As with the flowers, once you're familiar with the plant you'll have no trouble identifying elderberries.

Here are some plants with certain characteristics in common with elderberry. Some are highly poisonous, while others merely aren't elder (and may have other medicinal properties). Find images of these plants online, and pay attention to the different leaf patterns, arrangements of berries and flowers, and other distinguishing features, so you're sure what you've got is an elderberry.

Flowers that bear similarities to elderflowers:

Water Hemlock (*Cicuta virosa*)
Water hemlock is one of the most poisonous plants in North America, so it's an extremely important one for foragers to know. Also known as cowbane

---

3   Samuel Thayer, *Nature's Garden* (Birchwood, WI : Forager's Harvest Press, 2010), 401.

or poison parsnip, water hemlock has flowers that bear a passing resemblance to elderflowers, but it does not bear fruit. Note that water hemlock is *herbaceous*, meaning *it has no woody parts or bark like the elder.* So if you see a cluster of flowers and no bark, you do not have elder! Water hemlock has alternating rather than opposite compound leaves, and the flower head is rounded rather than flattened, with space between the individual inflorescences. *Conium maculatum*, also known as poison hemlock, grows more commonly in Europe. Be sure to learn what these plants look like and avoid them!

Red Elderberry (*Sambucus racemosa*)
There's some difference of opinion on the edibility of red elderberry, but many people experience severe stomach upset when they consume it, even cooked, so it's best to avoid. Native Americans used red elderberry for food and medicine. In my area, red elderberry flowers bloom and the red berries ripen a full month before *canadensis*. The flowerhead is pyramidal rather than flat and leaves are less toothed than black elderberry.

Hydrangea (*Hydrangea arborescens*)
A common foundation planting, white hydrangeas only resemble elderflowers from a distance. The most common white hydrangea flowerheads are rounded rather than flat; others are triangular or pyramidal in shape. Individual blossoms have heart-shaped petals. Compare images of the flowers online, and you'll have no worries about mistaking them. The rounded leaves are arranged in a very different pattern as well.

False Spirea (*Sorbaria sorbifolia*)
With a similar leaf pattern and tiny white flower clusters, the false spirea bears some resemblance to elder. The flowerheads are triangular, however, and the leaves contain more pairs of leaflets with more prominently veined leaves.

Cow Parsley (*Anthriscus sylvestris*)
Also known as wild chervil, wild beaked parsley, or keck, cow parsley is another *herbaceous* plant with a white flowerhead. The flower clusters are arranged in a more spread out manner, and the leaves resemble ferns.

Giant Cow Parsley (*Heracleum mantegazzianum*)
Also called giant hogweed, this *herbaceous* plant's sap is phototoxic, meaning that if it touches your skin and you expose that area to sunlight, you can get a severe and painful burn. It grows up to fourteen feet tall, has thick, bright green stems with purple blotches and white hairs, and can produce flowerheads over three feet in diameter.

Ground Elder (*Aegopodium podagraria*)
Also known as bishop's weed, goutweed, and snow-on-the-mountain, ground elder is not related to elderberry. An herbaceous plant commonly used as ground cover, it was once used medicinally for gout and arthritis. The stark difference in the leaf pattern from *Sambucus* makes ground elder easy to distinguish.

Plants that also produce dark berries:

Dwarf Elder (*Sambucus ebulus*)
Also known as danewort or dane weed, dwarf elder is the powerful emetic mentioned in Greek and Roman sources. Thayer notes that the *herbaceous* dwarf elder that is native to Europe may be found occasionally in North America. The berries, which do not droop when ripe, are considered toxic and reportedly taste terrible. The scent of the leaves has been described as "foetid." The flowerheads are not as flat and may have purple-tipped stamens. In France, says Bertrand Bouflet, the elderberry enthusiast behind La Maison du Sureau, most people confuse the dwarf elder (called *yéble* or *hièble* in French) with common elder (*S. nigra*) and mistakenly believe both are poisonous.

You may recall the historical medicinal uses of dwarf elder, used to induce vomiting. If that's not the effect you're after, if you see black berries that aren't drooping on an herbaceous plant, move on.

Virginia Creeper (*Parthenocissus quinquefolia*)
Virginia creeper is a vigorous climbing plant rather than a shrub. It has groups of five leaves arranged in a palm shape and produces clusters of berries that turn dark purple in summer.

Black Nightshade (*Solanum nigrum*)
There's some disagreement about the edibility of black nightshade, but besides their black berries, they don't have much in common with elderberries. They

grow on low, *herbaceous* plants with heart-shaped leaves and produce small clusters of berries. A related plant, called deadly nightshade (*Atropa bella-donna*) is, as the name implies, extremely toxic.

Red Osier Dogwood and Silky Dogwood (*Cornus sericea* and *Cornus amomum*)
Red osier dogwood and silky dogwood can grow in similar locations and have similar growth habits to elder. Pay particular attention to the different ways the leaves grow. Elder's compound and serrated leaves look quite different from the smoother leaves of the dogwood, which grow individually from the branch. Dogwoods' berries and flowers are larger, fewer, and spaced further from one another in berry clusters that tend to ripen later than elderberries. Berries of the red osier dogwood are white rather than dark purple.

Hercules' Club (*Aralia spinosa*)
Also known as devil's walking stick, prickly ash, or prickly elder, Hercules' club also has dark berries on red stems that ripen around the same time as elderberries. It grows in similar conditions and has somewhat similar leaves. The best way to identify Hercules' club is the dangerous thorns on its bark. (Elders do not have thorns.) Steve Brill writes, "If Hercules were to swat you on the butt with it, you'd take your meals standing for a very long time." He also warns that some people get a poison ivy–like rash from touching the bark.[4]

Pokeweed (*Phytolacca americana*)
Also known as pokeberry, ink berry, pigeonberry, poke salad, or just poke, poke-weed is an *herbaceous* plant with considerably larger, pea-sized berries that grow in long, thin clusters rather than the sprawling cymes of elderberries. Pokeberry leaves are simple and alternate in contrast to elderberry's compound, opposite leaves.

Chinese Privet (*Ligustrum sinense*)
The leaves of this invasive species are leathery and smooth rather than serrated. Privet has elongated flower and berry clusters rather than flat, round cymes. Flowers have four rather than five petals.

---

4   Brill, 57–8.

Arrowwood (*Viburnum dentatum*)

Arrowwood has white umbels of flowers that at first glance resemble elderflowers, but their simple, rounder leaves do not look like the pinnate leaflets of the elder. The purple berries arrowwood produces are reportedly edible but lack flavor.

Foraging Elderflowers and Elderberries

FORAGING ELDERFLOWERS

Elderflowers begin to bloom in late spring to early summer, depending on your region and the timing of spring weather. Bloom time occurs over a four- to six-week period, and berries begin to ripen roughly a month later.

Delicate elderflowers are best collected early in the day. Andrea Beddows, who manages Belvoir Farms' ninety acres of elderflower plantations in Lincolnshire, England, advises that "dry, pollen-rich flower is the most flavoursome and

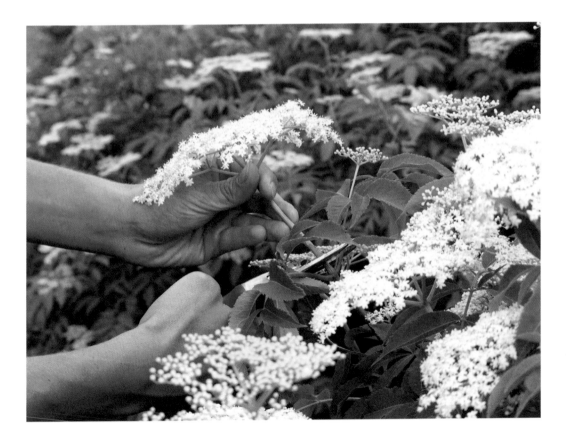

aromatic." She recommends picking early in the morning on a dry, sunny day and infusing or preserving your flowers as quickly as possible to preserve the best flavor.

Simeon Rossi, who uses large quantities of elderflowers for Loon Liquor's popular elderflower liqueur, says elderflowers may keep in the refrigerator for a day or two if you can't process them immediately.

To harvest elderflowers, carefully snip the stem of each flowerhead, keeping it upright if possible so the pollen doesn't fall off. Place heads in a clean paper bag or large box or basket. *Be sure to leave plenty of flowers on the plants, or you won't have any elderberries to harvest.*

Inspect carefully for bugs, which you should remove by hand. Resist the urge to wash your flowers, as you will rinse away the pollen, and with it the flavor and scent of elderflower.

The blossoms of some varieties of elderflower may be easier or more difficult to remove than others. Rossi warns that it takes hours to painstakingly remove all the flowers from the stems, which he finds impart a "chlorophyll-y" flavor that obscures the delicate fruitiness of the flower. He removes large numbers of blossoms efficiently using a clean plastic comb to rake off the tiny flowers with quick motions. We noticed as we worked our way through one of his three cases of flowers (enough to make about three hundred bottles of elderflower liqueur, requiring 10 to 12 hours of patient destemming) that this method left a fair number of flowers on the stem.

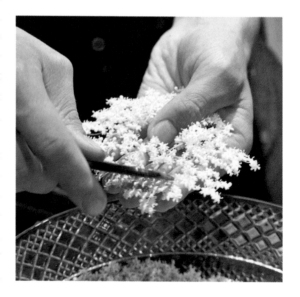

I tried slower motions and removed more flowers but also wound up with somewhat more stem in the bowl, which I then had to pick through and remove. But it also beat my hands up considerably less than the quick-rake method.

If you try the comb method, test out a couple different size combs to see what works for you. Since you're likely dealing with far smaller quantities, speed won't matter as much. You can also just pinch off the tiny flowers if you have a small number, but more of the precious pollen, the source of the scent and taste, wound up on my fingers this way.

FORAGING ELDERBERRIES

Once you've established you have the right plant, you'll be looking for blue-black clusters of berries starting about a month after flowering, usually toward the end of summer. The berries on each shrub will ripen over several weeks, so harvest only the fully-ripe clusters and leave the others until they're ready. You want to watch carefully, or you'll find that the birds have cleared the plants before you get any!

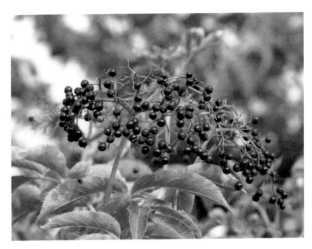

Samuel Thayer advises, "if you find a loaded elderberry bush late in the season, be skeptical. All elderberries are not equal. Birds know this, and they have a serious sweet tooth, often gleaning the last berry from a tasty tree before moving on to the insipid ones."[5] He recommends taste testing, but since most raw berries from *canadensis* shrubs don't have much flavor, this might work better with *cerulea* varieties.

Like the flowerheads, the berries on a given cluster may be in different stages of ripeness. While snipping a whole head saves time in the field, if you wind up with a bunch of under-ripe berries in the kitchen you've wasted some effort (and valuable food). If you find an unevenly ripe cluster, you can snip off the riper parts and leave the rest, or even pick off ripe berries individually. Really ripe ones can sometimes be knocked off into your container.

Pay close attention to when berries in your area begin to ripen, or you will lose virtually all of them to the birds. If you find shrubs stripped of berries, look for more bushes in shadier areas—which will likely ripen later—and you might

---

5   Thayer, 405.

spot some that haven't been picked over yet. If they're still red or green, be sure to come back every day or two so you can get them when they're ready.

To harvest, snip entire bunches of the ripest elderberries, rather than picking them individually. Fresh berries will keep in the refrigerator for a few days, but it's best to use, dry, or freeze them as soon as you can. When you're ready to process your berries, rinse well to remove insects and dust.

To de-stem your berries, remove them with a fork or your fingers, choosing only the ripest berries and discarding the green and reddish ones. This can be tedious work, but there are some tricks I learned from the pros to make it quicker. Some foragers prefer to freeze the bunches first as it can make removal considerably easier, but some (not all) find that this method results in more stems that you will then have to pick out. It's also harder to distinguish the ripe and less ripe berries once frozen. For large quantities of berries, freezer space can be an issue with this method as well.

I have also seen people recommend whacking the berry cluster against the side of a clean pail, which leaves the unripe berries on the stem. If you're processing a large number of berries, Terry Durham of River Hills Harvest elderberry farm, who has worked with the University of Missouri and Missouri State University Elderberry Improvement Project for over twenty years, recommends gently rubbing the berries against a screen made of ¼- to ⅜-inch stainless steel hardware cloth held over a colander or bucket. (He also designed a stainless-steel destemming tray for elderberries that he sells on his website.) Once you've removed the berries from the stem, he suggests submerging them in water. Unripe berries and stem fragments will float to the top and can be skimmed off. *Remember to remove all stems and twigs, as these contain compounds that can make you sick.*

Chapter 5 will cover what you need to know to prepare your elderberries and flowers safely and for maximum effectiveness.

CHAPTER 4

GROWING ELDERBERRY
IN THE HOME LANDSCAPE

"There should, of course, be an elder tree in every herb garden;
for have not herbs since time immemorial been under the protection of the
spirit of the elder tree?"
—Eleanour Sinclair Rohde, *A Garden of Herbs*, 1936[1]

If you don't have elderberries growing wild in your neck of the woods, cultivating elderberries in your garden is easy and rewarding. Even if you do have access to foraged berries, there are numerous reasons you might want to grow your own as well. First, you can select varieties that have traits you desire, such as sweeter fruit or more fragrant flowers. Even if you don't oth-

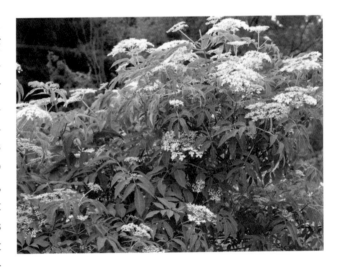

erwise grow food in your yard, elderberries are beautiful shrubs like many other common landscaping choices, but they offer the added benefit of delicious edible flowers and fruits. They're undemanding plants and offer food for wildlife as well as your family. Harvesting plenty of berries each season is even easier if you have shrubs in your own yard that you can watch for ripeness and protect from birds. Elder is a popular plant for hedgerows, as they grow quickly and form a thicket, great for borders of gardens or places where you want to create a living screen.

Elderberries benefit the home garden in a number of ways, aside from their magical protective powers. In *Edible Forest Gardens*, ecological designer David

---

1   Rohde, 11.

Jacke calls elderberry "a marvelous multipurpose plant," noting that in addition to their delicious berries and flowers, they provide "a valuable early-season nectar source for attracting specialist beneficial insects." He describes them as "low maintenance and widely adaptable. They thrive in wet areas most fruits cannot abide."[2] Because elderberries can tolerate the toxic juglones secreted by walnuts, they're often combined in permaculture guilds with these challenging trees. Permaculture expert Toby Hemenway notes elderberry's use as a "soil fumigant and pest repellant."[3] Permaculture design values plants that can serve additional purposes, so one that provides not only food for humans and wildlife, but also dye, wood crafts, and ingredients for homemade pesticides (see below, and recipe on page 182) checks an impressive number of boxes.

Elderberry shrubs will draw pollinators to your yard while they're in bloom, and if you don't mind sharing fruits with the birds, they should also attract plenty of feathered friends to enhance your birdwatching. Over forty species of bird are known to eat elderberries! Others rely on the insects that inhabit elders.

Maud Grieve included a number of ways to use elder in the garden in *A Modern Herbal*, including putting its notoriously stinky leaves to use as a pest repellent:

> The leaves have an unpleasant odour when bruised, which is supposed to be offensive to most insects, and a decoction of the young leaves is sometimes employed by gardeners to sprinkle over delicate plants and the buds of the flowers to keep off the attacks of aphids and minute caterpillars.

Elder leaves could also protect the gardener from attacks by insects:

> The leaves, bruised, if worn in the hat or rubbed on the face, prevent flies settling on the person. In order to safeguard the skin from the attacks of mosquitoes, midges, and other troublesome flies, an infusion of the leaves may be dabbed on with advantage.

---

2   David Jacke, *Edible Forest Gardens*, Volume One (Vermont: Chelsea Green, 2005), 320.
3   Toby Hemenway, *Gaia's Garden* (Vermont: Chelsea Green, 2009), 136.

Grieve also notes that "The leaves are said to be valued by the farmer for driving mice away from granaries and moles from their usual haunts." John Jeavons' popular *How to Grow More Vegetables* advises that cuttings from elderberries placed in gopher holes may repel them. Knowing the famed odor of Shakespeare's "stinking elder," I was surprised that I noticed no smell at all foraging our local elderberries. I then made a point to tear into *canadensis* leaves from numerous plants, and they all smelled, well, like leaves. Quite pleasant, really. The North American growers I spoke to confirmed that their *canadensis* leaves lacked the smell elders are famous for. You might need leaves from a *nigra* or dwarf elder if pest control is your goal.

French sources recommend a fermented concoction of *nigra* leaves to repel insects and rodents and mention that it may also help control fungal infections. If you'd like to try for yourself, instructions for making your own elder-leaf garden spray can be found at the end of the recipe section, page 182.

Cultivars to Consider

There are dozens of elderberry varieties to choose from. While it's possible to propagate new plants from a wild shrub, you won't have much information about the plant's disease resistance, productivity, and other attributes beyond what you can determine through your own observations. To know what you're planting in your home landscape, you may want to purchase cuttings or live plants that have been selected for various desirable characteristics. Andrew Thomas, a horticultural researcher at the University of Missouri, has been investigating elderberry varieties for twenty-three years and reports that there's been little breeding of elderberry. The named plants sold today have been propagated from wild cuttings of plants noted for their high yields, sweeter fruit, or resistance to pests.

Most elderberry cultivars are suited to planting zones 4 to 8, but you can find some varieties hardy to zone 3 or tolerant of the heat of zones 9 to 10.[4] It's likely cultivars bred from a variety native to your region—*canadensis* in the eastern and central US, *cerulea* in the west—will perform better for you than if you try to grow European elder in New Mexico, North Dakota, or Mississippi. Even a

4   Charlebois et al., 226. Charlebois has found plants growing in zone 2 as well, though the growing season may be too short to get fruit. naldc.nal.usda.gov/download/47014/PDF

plant of the same name, say *S. cerulea* or blue elderberry may vary widely in the conditions it's used to, which may be as different as the pacific northwest and Mexico. Likewise, the *Sambucus canadensis* that hails from Minnesota might not do well in your Florida garden or vice versa. Be sure if you're ordering cuttings or plants online that you check with the grower about how they have fared in climates like yours.

Brent Madding of 360 Farms cautions that local growing conditions can have a major impact on how your plants fare. Less than half the Bob Gordon elderberries he planted survived, and those that did produce fruit he describes as "unpalatable" because they're growing in an area dominated by sandstone rather than the limestone where their cultivar originated.

Trials of most European elderberry varieties in the American midwest—where it gets too hot in the south and too cold in the north—have tended to do poorly, and there hasn't been much research on their success in other parts of the country. If your climate closely resembles that of central Europe, you may

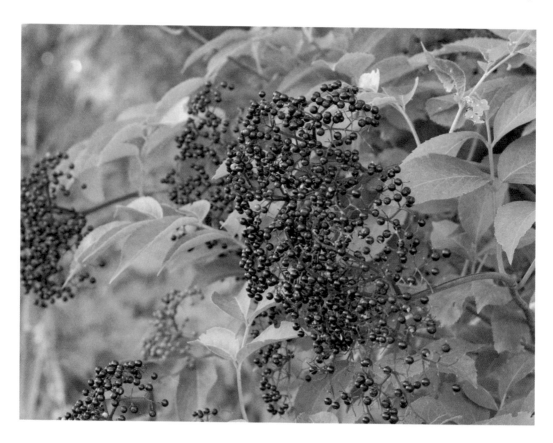

have better luck. But the growers I spoke to favor our native *canadensis* for its better-tasting and less-cyanogenic fruit, anyhow, so there's not much reason to try to grow a non-native variety, with one exception. One cultivar, Marge, has *nigra* lineage but outperformed native varieties in trials conducted at the University of Missouri.

Some elderberry cultivars reportedly produce better if there's more than one plant or more than one variety, though researchers say in most cases planting more than one variety isn't necessary.[5] There are advantages to getting multiple varieties, though, as you may find some do better in your specific growing conditions than others, and experts advise that plant diversity is just generally a good idea. In addition to improving the odds of a good yield, different cultivars will also extend your season for harvesting flowers and berries and provide a longer window for feeding pollinators.

Note that many elderberry varieties can get quite large, so you'll want to allow plenty of space. More compact cultivars might be better choices for the average home landscape, but even they will produce suckers and will need pruning to keep them from taking over.

On pages 74 and 75 you'll find selections that growers recommend for different purposes and growing conditions. Some are more readily available than others; you may need to search a bit to find some of the less common varieties. Plants sold by different vendors may have originated from different stock, so you'll find slightly different maximum heights and growing zones. The "ornamental" varieties listed here do bear fruit but generally yield less. (And those not listed as specifically ornamental are still beautiful!)

---

5   Charlebois et al., 223.

ELDERBERRY VARIETIES

Top choices for North American gardens in the Northeast and Midwest:

'Ranch'—A top recommendation from the growers I spoke with, Ranch is exceptionally adaptable, tolerating a range of conditions and poor soils better than many varieties. Durham reports that Ranch grows well from coast to coast, and in the coldest and warmest climates. These compact plants top out at 5 to 6 feet tall. Zones 3–8.

'Bob Gordon'—One of the most popular varieties among commercial growers, prized for its large, sweeter-than-average fruit. An especially productive plant, reaching 6 to 8 feet tall. Berry clusters can weigh up to two pounds. Zones 4–8.

'Marge'—Marge is one of the few European elderberries (*ssp. nigra*) that do well in North America. In a study at the University of Missouri, Marge outperformed American varieties, producing up to three times as much fruit and showing better disease resistance. Researchers found Marge to be "exceptionally robust and drought-resistant." Marge's berries are larger than most.[6] Marge can grow 6 to 12 feet tall, tending to grow larger in more temperate climates. Zones 3–10.

'Wyldewood'—A very productive variety known for its enormous flower heads. Later season than most, exceptionally cold-hardy. Grows 5 to 8 feet tall and wide. Zones 3–8.

'Oklahoma John'—Developed and propagated by Brent Madding of 360 Farms, Oklahoma John is a mutation of Wyldewood with double the production. It has larger berries than Wyldewood growing in very large clusters that are easier to de-stem. In warmer planting zones it will produce several additional flower heads down the cane. It came from clay soil near his farm, and is growing well for customers who have purchased it in a range of climates.

'York'—A more compact option that tops out at 6 feet tall and wide, York is a popular choice for home growers. It has larger berries than most, but some sources say they have lower sugar content and less flavor. Devon Bennett of Norm's Farms, however, thinks they're one of the most flavorful varieties. Said to be a good producer. Zones 3–8.

---

6   A. L. Thomas et al., "'Marge': A European Elderberry for North American Producers," *Acta Horticulturae* 1061 (2015): 191–199.

'Adams'—A larger plant, Adams grows 8 to 10 feet tall and wide and produces large flowerheads and berry clusters. Zones 3–9.

'Johns'—A publication from the University of Vermont's Center for Sustainable Agriculture says the berry clusters are exceptionally large, but the overall yield is less than Adams. Ten to 12 feet tall and wide. Zones 4–8.

'Nova'—This compact variety grows 6 feet tall and wide, producing good yields of large berries. Somewhat less cold-hardy than some other varieties. Zones 4–8.

For the Western United States:

Blue Elderberry—Blue elderberry has not gotten as much attention from growers developing cultivars, so you will mostly find them referred to as simply "blue elderberry" or *Sambucus cerulea*, though you may also see them called *'glauca,'* *'mexicana,'* or *'velutina.'* Plants named *mexicana* tend to be more drought-tolerant, having adapted to the arid conditions of the southwest. Growing 20 to 30 feet tall and wide, these are big trees that produce huge quantities of beautiful blue fruits, reported to be far tastier than *canadensis*. Its native range spans growing zones 6 through 10, and one seller reports hardiness to -20°F. Buying a plant from a local nursery will make it more likely it's suited to your garden's conditions.

Top choices for European gardens (or temperate North American gardens):

'Haschberg'—The most popular variety for European commercial production, Haschberg produces abundant, flavorful berries. Grows 6 to 8 feet tall. Zones 4–9.

'Samdal' and 'Samyl'—High-yielding Danish varieties that grow 6 to 8 feet tall but only 2 to 5 feet wide. Samyl is reported to have slightly better yields. Zones 3–8.

Ornamental varieties:

'Black Lace'—European variety, very ornamental with lacy dark purple foliage and pink flowers with a lemony scent, 6 to 8 feet tall and wide. Zones 4–7.

'Black Beauty'—European variety with purple foliage and pink flowers. One elderflower aficionado thinks Black Beauty's flowers may have a superior flavor to other varieties. 8 to 15 feet tall and 4 to 8 feet wide. Zones 4–8.

'Variegata'—European variety with, as the name suggests, variegated green and white leaves. Less productive than some, it grows up to 13 feet tall and 6 feet wide. Zones 4–10.

Siting and Soil

Choose a location with full sun for best yields, though you'll find plenty of wild elderberry shrubs doing quite well with partial shade. You'll still get berries in shadier locations, just not as many. Elderberries prefer well-drained, slightly acidic soil (pH 5.5 to 6.5) that's high in organic matter, but they're generally tolerant of poorer soils and grow well on marginal lands around farms.

Elderberries' shallow root systems mean they need consistent watering, about one to two inches per week, depending on what kind of soil they're planted in (and who you talk to). Elders don't like having what's referred to as "wet feet," so avoid placing them where water tends to pool. If you have heavy clay soil that doesn't drain well, you may want to grow them in raised beds, though some growers have found elderberry can handle poorly-drained soil and swamps. Very sandy soil will require amendment with organic matter to retain moisture and provide the nutrition plants need.

Be sure to leave enough space between plants to allow ample air flow. Though the potted plant you pick up at a nursery may be only a foot tall, it will need lots of room to grow. Remember, if its full width is eight feet, you'll need eight feet between plants so they can expand four feet in every direction, though some high-volume growers plant as close as four feet to make harvests more efficient. For best yields, plant within fifty feet of another elderberry.

Elderberry is perfect for the permaculture garden, serving multiple purposes. In addition to producing food and medicine for you, it attracts pollinators and provides food and habitat for wildlife. Permaculture design aims to make the most of garden space as well as inputs like water and fertilizer by growing plants in mutually beneficial arrangements called guilds. Though most people surround shrubs with grass, you can significantly increase the productivity of your garden by selecting plants that mutually benefit one another. Because elderberries need a moderate amount of nitrogen, underplanting your elderberry with nitrogen-fixing plants like clover can help nourish your elderberry and enhance soil microbiota. You can add other herbs you'll enjoy using medicinally and in cooking, such as lemon balm, mints, bee balm, violets, and thyme. In addition to the plentiful elder blossoms, the flowers of these useful and delicious herbs will provide a steady supply of food for pollinators, helping to increase yields in your garden.

Like elderberries, currants can tolerate the juglones put out by walnuts and hickories, so they are often planted alongside elderberries and can help extend your harvest of delicious and antioxidant-rich fruits. However, the elderberry growers I spoke with to advise mulching rather than underplanting to avoid competition for nutrients. If you do try underplanting, consider leaving some space around your elderberry shrub covered with mulch to ensure they get the nutrition they need.

Propagating Elderberry

There are numerous ways to obtain elderberry plants for your home garden. Which you choose will depend on your budget and tolerance for fuss. You can buy potted or bare-root plants online and at local nurseries, or obtain cuttings, either from wild plants, other gardeners, or nurseries.

CAN YOU GROW ELDER FROM SEED?

Though your elderberries will have thousands of seeds, planting elderberry from seed can be challenging, and most growers don't recommend it, in large part because there's no guarantee the resulting plant will have any of the desirable traits you noticed in the parent. If you find such challenges appealing and want to try, you'll need to do what's called "stratifying," which means giving your elderberry seeds a long chill (about twelve weeks) in your refrigerator before they will germinate in soil.

BUYING PLANTS

The simplest, but also the most expensive, way to get elderberry shrubs is buying potted plants at a nursery, where they will cost twenty to thirty dollars apiece. You may also order bare-root plants, which should cost somewhat less. Plan to purchase and plant in spring as growers often run out in the fall.

TRANSPLANTING RUNNERS OR ROOTS

Probably the easiest way for home gardeners to propagate elderberries is digging up one of the many runners elders send out and replant it in early spring before bud break as you would when you divide perennials in your garden. The plant that grows from it will be genetically identical to the mother plant, so choose one with characteristics you want. You can also take a 4- to 6-inch cutting from shallow roots while the plant is dormant in late winter. Cuttings should be about the diameter of a pencil and have three to five nodes. Place in growing media for 6 to 8 weeks and keep moist until roots develop before replanting in spring.

GROWING FROM CUTTINGS

You may recall from the folklore section the European tradition of planting elder twigs by graves, which would take root to show the departed was well. Elderberries grow readily from such cuttings, which can save you a good bit of money over buying nursery plants. Several growers sell cuttings online, but try to buy from somewhere with similar growing conditions to yours. A cutting from a farm in Georgia won't necessarily be happy at your Montana homestead, though several sellers of cuttings I spoke to report success from their customers in a variety of growing zones. You can also try taking a cutting from a neighbor's plant if it has characteristics you like. You're rolling the dice a bit taking from a wild-growing plant in your area, but if it's one you've seen that's doing well in conditions quite like your own and you have permission, you may want to try.

PROPAGATING PLANTS FROM CUTTINGS

According to Andrew Thomas, softwood cuttings are much more "involved" and "risky" than propagating from hardwood cuttings, and it's generally not recommended.

In contrast, says Byers, propagating elderberries from hardwood cuttings is "so easy." You can take your own hardwood cuttings or buy them from growers who do mail order, typically costing three to four dollars per cutting depending on the volume you order. Cuttings need cold weather to root, so they will be mailed between January and April, depending on your growing zone.

Planting and Care

It's always a good idea to test your garden soil before planting to identify nutrient deficiencies you should correct to help your plants thrive. Durham notes that soils often lack boron and sulphur, nutrients elderberries need. A soil test will also prevent adding unneeded nutrients, which can harm the plant and pollute waterways when it runs off.

After the danger of frost has passed in spring, prepare your site for transplanting by digging a hole two feet deep and two to three feet wide. Inspect the roots of the plant, which should be white or cream colored. If the plant is rootbound, with the roots spiraling around rather than reaching out, you should gently pull them loose, but do not spread them, counsels Brent Madding. Elderberry naturally wants to spread, and he says encouraging the plant to develop a dense root mat reaching further down into the soil will help it survive dry spells.

Durham recommends working in plenty of compost when you plant elderberries. In addition to adding valuable nutrients, compost encourages mycorrhizae, a complex network of underground fungi that greatly enhance the ability of plants to access nutrients in the soil. Use about 50 percent compost when you backfill your planting hole. Place the plant in your prepared hole with the top of the roots at or just below the level of the soil. Gently press the soil down and water thoroughly. Be sure to keep plants well-watered while they're getting established, 1 to 2 inches per week. Once established, these tough plants don't need much tending but will likely produce better with an annual application of fertilizer. Chris Patton, president of the Midwest Elderberry Cooperative, recommends an application of a 10-10-10 fertilizer when the plants begin to leaf out at a rate of a quarter pound per year of the plant, up to a pound per plant (in other words, ¾ pound for a 3-year-old plant, and a pound for any plant four years or older). Durham feeds his plants three times per year: 1) in spring, compost to nourish the soil and support the growth of the plant; 2) at flowering, a foliar feed such as compost tea; and 3) in fall after the berry harvest, a low-nitrogen, high phosphorus and potassium fertilizer.

After planting, mulch with 3 to 4 inches of wood chips or straw to prevent weeds from competing for nutrients. Ann Lenhardt says rotting hay and shredded bark mulch work well, but notes that hay breaks down more quickly and needs replacing more often. Pull out any weeds carefully to avoid damaging roots.

The first growing season, you should remove all the flowers (and make lots of tea, mead, champagne, and syrup!) to prevent the plant from putting its energy into fruit production. You want that energy to go to establishing a strong root system instead. You can start harvesting some fruit the second season. Each elderberry shrub can produce 10 to 15 pounds of fruit each year after the second or third year.

PRUNING

Though in the wild, elderberry shrubs go unpruned except by high winds and wildlife, in the home landscape you'll want to keep your elderberries pruned for several reasons. Elderberry shrubs will sucker and try to take over a larger area, so pruning will prevent them from crowding out other plants and help your shrubs maintain a tidier appearance. In the case of larger varieties, you will also have an easier time harvesting if you keep the plants smaller. Additionally, pruning increases airflow, which can help to prevent disease. Pruning can also encourage new canes to grow, creating a more productive plant.

No pruning is necessary in the first two growing seasons. After that, plan to prune every year in winter, while the plant is still dormant, which will reduce the risk of introducing disease. Using clean, sharp shears, prune any broken or dead canes. You need to know before you prune whether your variety of elderberry produces fruit on first-year or older canes. For varieties fruiting on first year canes, some growers recommend cutting all canes to ground level annually or every other year, which will encourage the plant to produce fewer but larger berry clusters that will ripen more evenly. If your variety does not fruit on first-year canes, prune canes more than three years old, which will not produce as much fruit as younger canes. Clean pruners after use and destroy any infected canes to discourage the spread of disease.

DISEASES AND PESTS

As native plants adapted to local growing conditions, elderberries in general aren't prone to many insect pests or diseases, though there are some to keep an eye out for.

Powdery Mildew

Some home growers have problems with powdery mildew, a fungal disease that affects many garden plants, especially towards the end of the seasons. If you spot powdery mildew on your elders' leaves, prune the affected stems and destroy them. You can treat the plant with a neem-based spray, which may also be used to control a number of other common pests and diseases. Powdery mildew tends to form on leaves in persistently wet conditions, so watering at the base of the plant rather than from above is an important prevention strategy. Allowing enough space for good air circulation will also help prevent powdery mildew.

Verticillium Wilt

An extremely destructive fungus, verticillium wilt will cause leaves to yellow and branches to die. Once a plant is infected it can't be saved, so you need to dig up the plant. The disease remains in the soil, so you shouldn't plant anything in the same spot that's susceptible to the disease, such as tomatoes, strawberries, mint, or potatoes. Likewise, it's best not to plant your elderberries where these crops have recently grown. Solarizing your soil (covering with plastic sheeting for a month or more in summer) may kill off the fungus.

Thread Blight

Thread blight is a fungus that causes leaves to wilt, curl, and brown. The fungus is a white thread-like fiber on canes. Remove infected branches and prune to encourage airflow and sunlight penetration.

Tomato Ringspot Virus

Tomato ringspot virus weakens the plant and may kill it over time. A yellowish ring may appear on the leaves. Avoid planting elderberry where members of the nightshade family (*Solanaceae*), which can harbor tomato ringspot virus, have recently grown. Examples include tomatoes, potatoes, eggplants, and peppers.

Leaf Spot

Leaf spot may be caused by different types of fungus and occurs in very wet weather. Spots may be brown, yellow, or purple, and can cause the leaf to fall from the plant. Remove all infected leaves and branches, and avoid overhead watering.

Elderberry Borers, Cane Borers, Borer Beetles

These insects burrow through the stems of the plant and kill it. If you see wilting tips and find that the cane is hollow, cut off and destroy affected canes.

Eriophyid Mites

Eriophyid mites cause leaves to crinkle and cup. The University of Vermont's elderberry guide advises that "While the damage may look awful, most plants can tolerate the damage and using pesticides can actually make infestations worse." They recommend pruning out infected canes.

Spotted Wing Drosophila (SWD)

Chris Patton of the Midwest Elderberry Growers Cooperative reports that spotted wing drosophila (SWD), which has been ravaging regional small fruit crops in recent years, may also prove problematic for elderberries. We've had SWD in my area for many seasons now, and I've seen them destroy entire crops of raspberries and juneberries, which become squishy and rotten as they ripen. The elderberries I've collected, even on a farm with SWD, have not been detectably infected. Fine mesh netting (less than 1 mm) can be placed over the bush and anchored to the ground to exclude SWD. It has the added advantage of keeping out Japanese beetles and birds. One grower has also tried using nylon footie socks around berry clusters. Patton recommends neem oil sprays and homemade traps made with soda bottles and kombucha as a lure. The Midwest Elderberry Cooperative has lots more information about controlling SWD on their website.

Japanese Beetles

A familiar sight to home gardeners, Japanese beetles can wreak havoc on many garden plants, elderberry included. They love a number of perennial food plants, so those of us with permaculture gardens will find them attracted to our grapes, plums, apples, and raspberries, as well as to a number of common tree species and annual garden favorites. They appear quickly in large numbers and can defoliate a plant, which will have a negative impact on your berry crop.

The easiest way to control Japanese beetles is handpicking them into a container of soapy water, where they will drown. They're very easy to knock off the leaves into a bucket, especially in the morning and evening. The key is to start managing them as soon as you notice them so they don't have a chance to multiply.

Other pests and diseases can sometimes affect elderberries, including sawflies, rust, aphids, and thrips, but I doubt you'd like to read about all of them![7] If something looks amiss with your elderberry, your best bet is to call your local extension service for support.

Most home growers have few problems with these tough plants, so don't expect that you'll need to expend too much energy defending them from attack. Remember, they've got a reputation as a defender of gardens!

---

7   More information in Charlebois et al., 235–8.

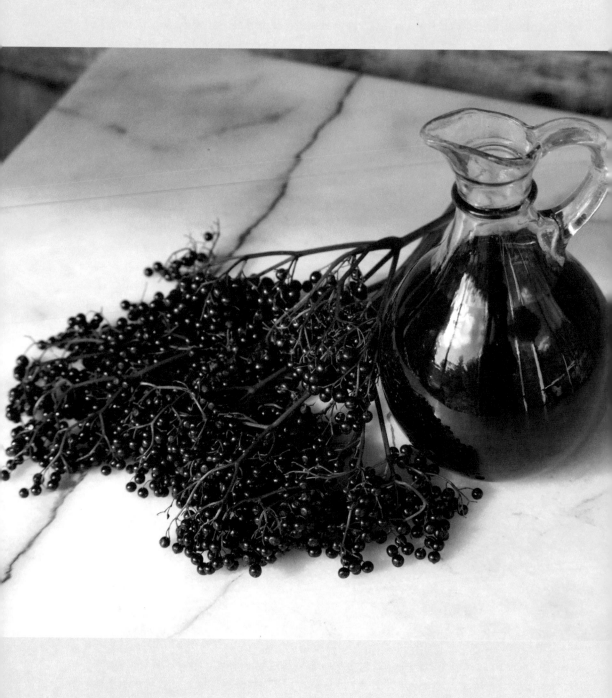

CHAPTER 5

PRESERVING AND PREPARING ELDERBERRIES AND ELDERFLOWERS

Elderberry Ketchup, for Fish Sauce—Pick a pint of ripe elderberries from the stalks, and put them into an earthen jar. Pour over them a pint of boiling vinegar, and let them remain in a cool oven all night. Strain the liquor from the berries without squeezing them, and put it into a saucepan with an ounce of shallots, a blade of mace, an inch of whole ginger, a tea-spoonful of cloves, and a tea-spoonful of peppercorns.
—*Cassell's Dictionary of Cookery*, 1892

What Parts Do We Eat?

We eat only the flowers and berries. Leaves, stems, roots, and bark are not considered safe to consume, though historically some were used in tea, often as an emetic (i.e., they can make you vomit). Most elder aficionados I've come across don't worry much about some tiny bits of the thinnest parts of the stem getting into their syrup or jam, but do your best to pick out as much stem material as possible. Though many people eat raw elderberries without problems, most sources advise cooking to break down the compounds that cause stomach upset. Some people are more sensitive than others to the seeds even when the berries are cooked, so don't eat a lot of them until you know if you're one of them. Rosalee de la Forêt says she's heard "countless times" that people have gotten very ill from consuming elderberry powder, which contains pulverized seeds (likely *nigra*). If you skipped the "Cautions" section in Chapter 2 (page 36), please go give it a read before preparing large quantities of elderberry.

Remember that the leaves have been used to make external preparations for soothing cuts and bruises and repelling insects. You'll also find a recipe at the end of the book for an Elder Leaf Salve for wounds, burns, and sprains (page 178).

Preserving Fresh Elderflowers and Elderberries

After all that work collecting elderflowers and elderberries, you want to preserve your harvest! Some can be transformed into syrups, tinctures, and syrups right away, but you'll probably want to "put up" some for future use. Both berries and flowers should be kept in the refrigerator if you won't be processing them immediately, as they start to deteriorate quite quickly at room temperature.

Maud Grieve cautions,

The flowers are not easily dried of good colour. If left too late exposed to the sun before gathering, the flowers assume a brownish colour when dried, and if the flower bunches are left too long in heaps, to cause the flowers to fall off, these heaps turn black. If the inflorescence is only partly open when gathered, the flower-heads have to be sifted more than once, as the flowers do not open all at the same time. The best and lightest coloured flowers are obtained at the first sifting, when the flowers that have matured and fallen naturally are free from stalks, and dried quickly in a heated atmosphere ...

Most pharmacopoeias specify that dark brown or blackish flowers should be rejected. This appearance may be due to their having been collected some time after opening, to carelessness in drying, or to having been preserved too long.

Brent Madding (whose farm focuses on elderflowers) emphasizes the importance of drying elderflowers *without* added heat. He recommends drying the flowers on their stems, preferably on a screen, to encourage airflow and preserve their color. When fully dry, remove the flowers from the stems and place in an airtight container.

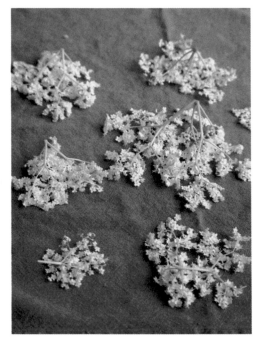

You'll be thrilled to have a big jar of dried elderflowers once cold season rolls around, but don't dry them all. You want fresh ones to make syrups, and you can also have some fun infusing vinegars, making tinctures, and baking with them. Depending on the plants you have access to, you'll likely have several weeks to gather flowerheads and try different recipes. A little jar of dried flowers or some elderflower vinegar make wonderful homemade gifts for friends and family.

Preserving the berries takes a little more effort. One of the easiest and most effective ways to preserve seasonal goodies like fresh fruit is dehydrating. Unlike canning, dehydrating takes virtually no skill or knowledge, and a decent dehydrator is a pretty small investment. Dehydrating is as simple as laying out fresh berries on the drying trays and turning the machine on for a few hours. Terry Durham says most commercially dried berries are frozen first, and much of the juice runs out of the berries. If you dry your own berries from fresh, you'll likely get more of their flavor and medicinal properties in the finished product.

It's easier to leave the berries on the stem to dehydrate and remove them once they've dried. Berries can be dried at 125 to 135°F. Depending on your berries and climate, it can take 4 to 15 hours to dry them completely. Check them after four hours, especially if your berries are small. If you live in a dry climate, you can try drying berries outdoors on a screen covered with netting to protect them from birds and insects, or in a solar dehydrator. Some people use their cars as solar dehydrators as well. Durham highly recommends freeze-drying if you have a home freeze-dryer, as these berries are "a whole different world" in terms of flavor.

Like other herbs in your kitchen, dried elderberries and elderflowers will lose their potency and flavor over time. Keep them in an airtight container away from light and heat, and try to use them within a year or so.

Another easy way to preserve berries is in your freezer—a good idea if you plan to make recipes calling for fresh berries. To freeze, put your cleaned berry clusters on a cookie sheet or in a bag in the freezer for a few hours before destemming and storing in a container or freezer bag. Note that, as with other frozen foods, the nutrients degrade over time. One study found that elderberries lost much of their anthocyanin content after months in the freezer, some varieties more than others. After nine months of storage, some varieties maintained less than a third of their original anthocyanins.[1]

Some people juice their elderberries, but since juicers may also extract compounds from seeds that you might not want to consume without heating, heating berries and straining the solids may be safer. For simple extraction on the

---

1   Johnson et al. Bob Gordon retained nearly all its original anthocyanin content after three months and more than half after nine. In contrast, the sample of Adams II they tested had only 42 percent at three months and only 18 percent after nine months of freezer storage.

stovetop, Durham recommends first freezing your berries to help break down cell walls, then placing them in a pot with a very small amount of liquid to thaw over low heat. Their juice will release easily, and then you can strain out the seeds and skins, the parts more likely to give sensitive people trouble. Steam juicing is another option to consider.

Fermenting is another popular option, and you'll find recipes for elderberry wine, elderflower mead, and kombucha in the Elderberry and Elderflower Drinks recipe section beginning on page 149.

Now that your pantry and freezer are stocked with elderberries, let's get cooking!

Elderberry and Elderflower Kitchen Creations

Readily available and easily harvested, elderberries and elderflowers have a long history of culinary use. Though you may have only encountered elder-berries in medicinal syrups, home cooks have been dishing up flavorful pies, sauces, wines, and jams for cen-turies. The earliest surviving European cookbook, *De re Coquinaria (On the Subject of Cooking)*, thought to date from the first century AD, includes a recipe for elderberry custard:

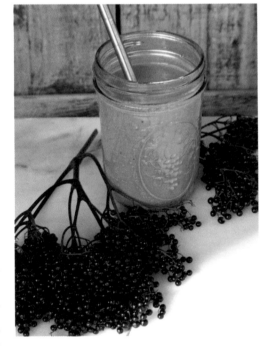

Elderberry Custard or Pie *Patina De Sambuco*

A dish of elderberries, either hot or cold, is made in this manner. Take elderberries wash them; cook in water, skim and strain. Prepare a dish in which to cook the custard, crush 6 scruples of pepper with a little broth; add this to the elderberry pulp with another glass of broth, a glass of wine, a glass of raisin wine and as much as 4 ounces of oil. Put the dish in the hot bath and stir the contents. As soon as it is getting warm, quickly break 6 eggs and whipping them, incorporate them, in order to thicken the fluid. When thick enough sprinkle with pepper and serve up.[2]

Centuries later, the ever-increasing number of cookbooks circulating as literacy rates rose and printing costs fell often included recipes calling for elderflowers and elderberries. Elderflower vinegar was a kitchen staple, and home-brewed elderberry wine remained a standard. Some eighteenth- and nineteenth-century cookbooks offered recipes for elder shoots, pickled elder buds, and elderberry "ketchup."

Moerman's *Native American Ethnobotany* records numerous culinary uses for elder among tribes across the continent. In addition to scores of medicinal uses, many tribes ate the berries raw, mashed them into dried cakes, or dehydrated them for winter. The Cherokee and Pima used elderberries for wine, pies, and jelly, for example, and the Iroquois and Cahuilla made sauces. The Dakota, Pawnee, and Omaha used elderflowers for tea.[3]

Receipt Book of John Nott, 1723:

TO PICKLE ELDER BUDS.—Put the Buds into Vinegar, season'd with Salt, whole pepper, large mace, lemon-peel, let them have two or three walms over the Fire; then take them out and let the Buds and Pickle both cool, then put the Buds into your Pot and cover them with the Pickle.

TO PICKLE ELDER TOPS.—Break the Tops of young Sprouts of Elder, about the middle of April, six inches long, let them have half a dozen walms in boiling Water, then drain them; make a pickle of wine water, salt, and bruised pepper, put them into the Pickle, and stop them up close.[4]

Eighteenth-century cooks regularly incorporated elderberry and elderflower into their culinary creations. Eliza Smith's popular 1727 cookbook, *The Compleat Housewife* includes recipes for pickled elder shoots ("A Pickle in imitation of Indian Bamboe"), several wines using berries and flowers, elderflower beer, a cure for the "Joint Evil" using fresh elder leaves—which will work "when

---

2   *De re Coquinaria,* English translation by Joseph Dommers Vehling, gutenberg.org/files/29728/29728 -h/29728-h.htm

3   Moerman, 512–15.

4   Quoted in Eleanour Sinclair Rohde, *Garden of Herbs* (London: P.L. Warner, 1921), 60.

all other remedies have failed"—as well as several other elder-based remedies.[5] Elizabeth Moxon's 1741 *English Housewifery* includes recipes for elderberry and elderflower wine, as well as pickled elder buds.[6] In a 1769 volume called *The complete English cook, or Prudent housewife*, Catharine Brooks also includes a recipe for elderberry wine and explains how to use elder leaves to treat sores and dropsy.[7] Susanna Carter's 1772 *The Frugal Housewife* names elderflower vinegar as one of "the best things to give a sauce tartness."[8]

Juliet Corson, a leading nineteenth-century cooking educator, columnist for the *New York Times,* and founder of the New York School of Cookery, promoted elder as a source of frugal and delicious ingredients. Her 1888 book *Family Living on $500 a Year: A Daily Reference-Book for Young and Inexperienced Housewives* advised foraging for elder shoots and making other creative uses of the elder: "Elder shoots, when they first appear, are good; as they grow a little they can be cooked like asparagus; the green buds salted are a substitute for capers; and even the flowers are made into pancakes." She does not bother going into detail about using elder for wine, she says, because "Elderberry wine is too well known to need recalling to country-bred folks."[9]

The 1892 edition of *Cassell's Dictionary of Cookery*, "containing about nine thousand recipes," has a page devoted to the uses of elder that includes recipes for elderberry wine, brandy, and rob, elderberry ketchup, elderflower vinegar, and pickled elder tops.[10] Elderflowers and elder vinegar are also called for in several additional recipes.

Elderberry was a common additive to grape wines to give them better body and flavor and was also used to counterfeit expensive wines like port or claret. Maud Grieve comments,

> Judiciously flavoured with vinegar and sugar and small quantities of port wine, Elder is often the basis of spurious 'clarets' and 'Bordeaux.' . . . Cheap port is often faked to resemble tawny port by the addition of

5   Eliza Smith, *The Compleat Housewife* (London: E. S. Smith, 1727), 240, 330.

6   Elizabeth Moxon, *English Housewifery* (Leeds: Thomas Wright, 1790).

7   Catharine Brooks, *The Complete English Cook; or, Prudent Housewife* (London: Jay Cooke, 1769).

8   Susanna Carter, *The Frugal Housewife; or, the Experienced Cook* (London: T. Hughes, 1826), 63.

9   Juliet Corson, *Family Living on $500 a Year: A Daily Reference-Book for Young and Inexperienced Housewives* (New York: Harper, 1888), 131.

10 *Cassell's Dictionary of Cookery* (London: Cassell, 1892), 203.

Elderberry juice . . . but as the berries possess valuable medicinal properties, this adulteration has no harmful results.

She relates the story of an American sailor who found that "old, dark-red port
was a sure remedy for rheumatic pains." His physician researched his claim and
learned "that while genuine port wine has practically no anti-neuralgic properties, the cheap stuff faked to resemble tawny port by the addition of elderberry
juice often banishes the pain of sciatica and other forms of neuralgia."

In the twentieth century, many commonly-available cookbooks included recipes using elderberries and elderflowers. Though the 1997 "New" *Joy of Cooking*
contained only a quick mention of elderberries ("No other fruit will give an apple
pie more verve"), prior editions included several elderberry recipes. The 1964
edition had a recipe for elderberry jam and mentioned using elderberries in
tisanes, while the 1946 edition suggested using elderflowers in pancakes or making elderflower fritters by dipping whole umbels in batter and deep frying. The
long-awaited 2019 update came out just as I was finishing this book, and I was
intrigued to see elderflowers reappear as a possible fritter ingredient, though the
suggestion to add elderberries to apple pie was gone. The 1972 *New York Times
Heritage Cookbook* included recipes for elderberry blossom wine and elderberry
chutney, and a 1946 Kerr canning booklet had a recipe for elderberry "catsup." As
recently as 2001 the well-known culinary encyclopedia *Larousse Gastronomique*
included recipes for elderflower wine and fritters, as well as for boiled elder
shoots, to be served warm with gravy, cream, or butter, or cold with a vinaigrette.

In many parts of the world, elder products never went out of fashion. The
syrup made from elderflowers is added to soft drinks across Europe. Coca Cola
launched an elderflower and lemon flavor under its Fanta label, though some
claim it contains no actual elderflower. Numerous British grocery store chains
have a house-brand elderflower soda, and Belvoir Fruit Farms' popular elderflower cordials can be found all over the world. At one time Trader Joe's made
a lemon and elderflower soda, and SodaStream created an elderflower syrup
for adding to home-carbonated water. Ikea also regularly stocks an elderflower
syrup (*saft fläder*) that's delicious in seltzer.

Elderflower liqueur, the best-known brand of which is St. Germain, has
become known as "bartender's ketchup," and is often added to numerous mixed
drinks to give them a little sparkle. (You'll find some cocktail inspiration in the
recipe section beginning on page 149.)

The Italian liqueur sambuca is often served neat with three coffee beans meant to represent health, happiness, and prosperity or seven meant to represent the seven hills of Rome. *Food and Wine* magazine has called sambuca "the unsung hero of your liquor cabinet," working beautifully in cocktails.

Elder enjoyed a bump in the culinary media when Meghan Markle chose elderflower as the flavor for her royal wedding cake in 2018. Articles explained elderflower to unfamiliar audiences, while numerous magazines and newspapers printed recipes for elderflower cake. Elderflower grower Brent Madding told me he was inundated with calls from people looking to buy elderflower syrup for their own confectionary creations and elderflowers for their wedding bouquets.

Cooking with Elderberry and Elderflower

When I first tried baking with fresh elderberries, I was disappointed to find that I really couldn't taste them. Numerous muffins, pancakes, and baked oatmeals had no detectable flavor of elderberry. I was perplexed, as I'd seen numerous enthusiastic recipes for elderberry baked goods of all sorts. Then I found this comment by influential proponent of wild foods Euell Gibbons in his classic *Stalking the Wild Asparagus*:

> As fresh-cooked fruit the elderberry has little to recommend it. In the course of my research, I tried numerous recipes for pies, sauces, and fruit soups, and found them all pretty nauseous mixtures.[11]

I find this overstates the case a bit for the berries I was using, which were merely bland, not in the least nauseating or "rank," another way he describes them. Gibbons goes on to say that "dried elderberries are a different matter entirely." I found that cooking down the fresh berries made a perfectly tasty jam, and Ashley Adamant, who blogs about foraged foods at Practical Self Reliance and contributed the Elderberry Tarts recipe (page 142), also thought a good simmer greatly improved the flavor of berries. She reports that dried berries worked well in her tarts and pie, though I've found the rehydrated dried berries too crunchy for things like muffins and oatmeal since they don't steep in juice the way they do for a pie. But they do work, so if you don't mind a little crunch and

---

11   Euell Gibbons, *Stalking the Wild Asparagus* (Brattleboro, VT: Alan C. Hood & Company, 1962), 92.

all you have are dried berries, maybe try rehydrating a few to experiment with the next time you bake. Just eat in moderation, as the vast majority of dried berries you can buy are *nigra*, which contain more cyanogenic glucosides than the *canadensis* berries.

Wild food expert Samuel Thayer finds the flavor of the blue elderberry (*cerulea*) far superior to the *canadensis*: "I am convinced that if the two grew together, almost everybody would ignore the American Elder. But considering the price of airfare, I suspect that we easterners will keep on using what we have and calling it good enough."[12] Flavor will vary widely among plants, and be influenced by growing conditions like soil and weather. The intensity of the flower flavor can vary significantly as well. Chris Patton told me that the U.K.-born secretary-treasurer of Patton's Midwest Elderberry Cooperative "had to cut his elderflower wine recipe in thirds" when he used midwestern elderflowers because they are so much more potent than those he grew up with.

The flavor and scent of elderflower products from Europe differs noticeably from those growing here in Minnesota. Our local elderflowers are lightly floral, and the syrup made from them very subtle. The bottled syrup from Ikea, in contrast, has a prominent smell and flavor of lychee completely absent in our local flowers. St. Germain, the elderflower liqueur from France, is also known for its strong lychee flavor. When I opened a sealed bag of dried *nigra* flowers I purchased, I was hit with a wave of lychee smell completely unlike the scent of those I gathered and dried myself.

Sensory scientist Alice Jones, who has worked with elderflowers in Europe professionally for over a decade, recently toured numerous North American elderberry farms to learn more about cultivation practices. Jones describes the flavor of the *canadensis* elderflower as "very sweet and vanilla-ey" in contrast to the European varieties, which have a "more citrusy" flavor profile. She also found that the flowers growing in New England had far less fragrance than those she sampled in the midwest. However, she explained to me, flavor is a very individual thing, and people will "perceive flavors in different ways depending on their genetics, so what I taste is not the same as what you experience." Expectations also play an important role in determining flavor, she says.

Whatever their scent, fresh elderflower is definitely what you want for most recipes, adding a magical and fragrant fresh flavor. But dried elderflowers can

---

12 Thayer 405

work as well, especially if you're just adding small quantities to baked goods for extra nutrition and herbal goodness. Dried flowers are also perfectly fine for tinctures and teas.

SUBSTITUTIONS FOR FOOD ALLERGIES

Grain-free
Substitute your favorite gluten-free mix or add elderberries to gluten-free recipes calling for blueberries. I've found a little lemon juice or lemon zest helps bring out their flavor if you're adapting a non-elderberry recipe.

Nut-free
Omit nuts or substitute sunflower seeds.

Dairy-free
Substitute your favorite nut milk (cashew, almond, coconut, or other dairy alternative) for milk and coconut yogurt for dairy yogurt.

Vegan
If gummies look appealing but the animal-based gelatin isn't for you, you can try using agar powder, though it's reportedly more finicky to use.

For baked goods, substitute maple syrup for honey, nut or alternative milks for dairy, and chia or flax "eggs" for eggs.

USEFUL TOOLS AND EQUIPMENT

Mason jars: Handy for tincturing, storing dried herbs, and steeping sun tea, a variety of mason jars can serve multiple uses in the budding herbalist's kitchen.

Dropper bottles: If you'll be making tinctures, a small number of dropper bottles will make serving up the right amounts easier.

Tea strainer: An infuser cup or teapot with a built-in strainer can simplify brewing teas and infusions. I use infuser cups for single servings and a quart-size tea pot for bigger batches.

Nut milk bag or cheesecloth: These help strain tiny herb particles, which can escape through the holes of a standard mesh strainer. I recommend a nut milk bag, which is washable and durable and can also be used for making delicious homemade nut milks.

Kitchen scale: Useful for those new to working with herbal remedies, it can help ensure you're adding the amounts called for, since herbs can vary quite a bit when measured by volume. Also helpful for all the European recipes for elder you'll find online using weight rather than volume measurements.

Using Elderflower and Elderberry in Recipes

There's an elderberry recipe for everyone, from a simple tea to homemade lozenges, a great replacement for cough drops. For little ones, you can add a stick and voilà!—you have a cough-busting, immune-boosting lollipop. I've combed the internet, historical cookbooks, and herbal guides to find these innovative, healing, and tasty recipes to help you get the most out of your elderberries.

I suspect many readers already or soon will enjoy foraging remedies for their herbal arsenal, so I've included several recipes with additional ingredients you can forage as well. When you've made the ones that appeal to you, head over to Pinterest and prepare to be stunned by all the intriguing and delicious things people are doing with elderberries and elderflowers!

A word on ingredients:
Those of us seeking more natural ways to support health tend to find numerous ways the modern world makes that difficult. I'm talking about pesticides, industrial chemicals, and artificial flavors and colors. Do yourself a favor and choose organic ingredients whenever possible and use only water from a high-quality filter to remove the astonishing number of contaminants in most public water supplies.

Likewise, what we're learning about plastic packaging's effects on our health (as well as the environment) means you should avoid it whenever you can. Buy foods in glass or paper whenever possible, and try to steer clear of ingredients in metal cans, since most are lined with some kind of plastic.

Lastly, as we've learned about the negative effects of sugar and processed food on our health, more of us are turning to whole foods. Especially since elderberries' most prized superpower lies in their ability to support our immune system, turning them into junk food seems counterproductive. If you're consuming elderberry often, I recommend using the base (rather than a sweetened syrup) added to smoothies or diluted in water as a tea. Though you will find some sweets and treats in the pages that follow, I've generally prioritized whole grains and less sugary recipes over highly-sweetened ones made with refined ingredients.

Happy cooking!

ELDERBERRY AND ELDERFLOWER RECIPES

PART I:
PREPARATIONS FOR IMMUNE SUPPORT

Elderflower Tea or Infusion

This light, floral tea has traditionally been used for treating colds and respiratory illness. Using fresh flowers makes a lighter, greener-tasting tea. The dried flowers brew up with a bit more depth and intense floral flavor, which I think is tasty enough to drink even if you're not treating a cold. See note below about making an infusion for treating colds and fevers. **Makes 1 cup**

2–3 teaspoons dried elderflowers (or about 2–3 tablespoons if using fresh blossoms)
8 ounces boiling water

In an infuser cup or teapot, add elderflowers and boiling water.

Steep at least 10 minutes, longer if possible.

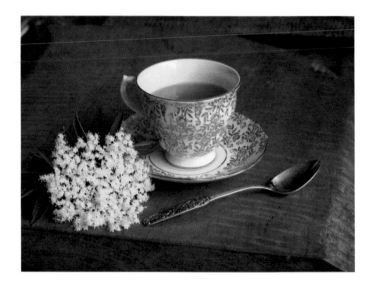

Notes:

- You can make a stronger infusion for acute situations, 1–3 tablespoons dried elderflowers per cup of water, steeped for several hours or overnight. To serve, warm it by diluting with a little hot water and drink throughout the day.
- Matthew Wood cautions fresh elderflowers may be harder on the stomach, so use dried flowers if that is a concern.
- An anti-inflammatory and diaphoretic, elderflower is a go-to herbal remedy for fever and seasonal allergies. Combine with peppermint and/or yarrow for colds and fever, or nettle for allergies. It also has relaxing properties and can be combined with chamomile for a lovely bedtime tea.

Elderberry Tea

Elderberry tea is probably the simplest way to enjoy elderberries, requiring nothing more than boiling water and dried elderberries. It's likely not the best way to maximize the medicinal power of elderberries, but sometimes it's all we're up for, and something is usually better than nothing! If you have time, simmering your berries to make an elderberry decoction (next recipe) will extract more of the medicinal compounds, while deactivating the ones people worry about. But don't sweat it if you don't have time, and enjoy this fruity brewed tea on occasion instead. **Makes 1 cup**

1 teaspoon dried elderberries
8 ounces boiling filtered water

In an infuser cup or teapot, add elderberries and boiling water. Steep at least 10 minutes, longer if possible, and up to 8 hours, to extract as much as possible from the elderberries. You can re-brew berries for a weaker second cup of tea.

Double Elder Tea

Double the power of elder by combining an infusion of the flowers with a decoction of the berries in this fruity and floral tea. It works best with a spiced syrup, but you can make it with base or plain syrup as well. **Makes 1 cup**

1 cup boiled filtered water
1 tablespoon dried elderflower
2 tablespoons Simple Elderberry Syrup (page 102) (or base plus honey to taste)

Infuse elderflowers in boiling water, at least 10 minutes and up to several hours.

Add elderberry syrup and serve warm, diluted with water if desired.

Notes:
- This recipe makes an intensely-flavored drink and would give you a pretty big dose of elderberry if you drank it all at once. Because it's most useful to take often, it's a good idea to dilute with hot water and sip throughout the day.

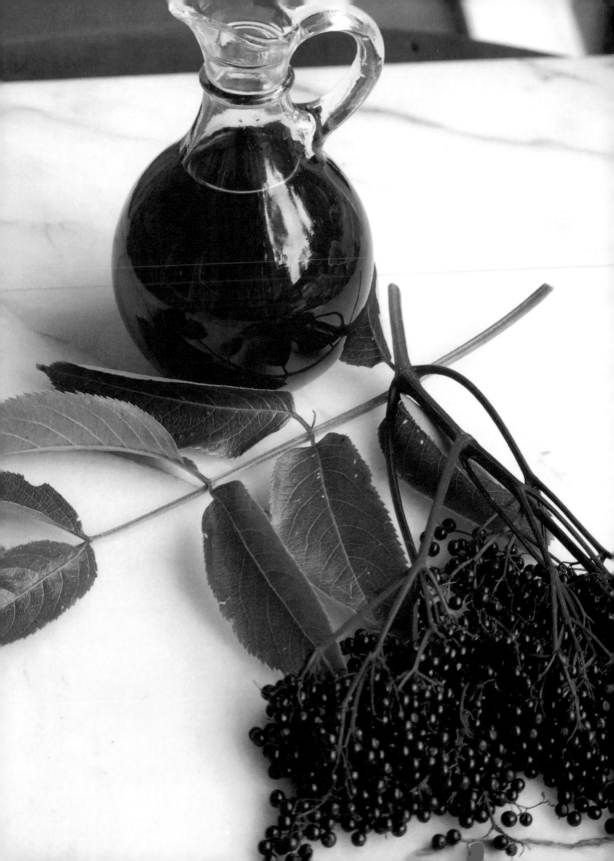

Elderberry Base (Decoction)

Just elderberries simmered in water, this base can be kept on hand for adding to drinks or turning into a more potent tea than if you simply pour water over the berries. Elderberry base won't keep as long as syrup made with honey (which acts as a preservative), but it's good to have for recipes where you might not want additional sweetener, like lemonade or cocktails. It's also a smart replacement for elderberry syrup if what you're after is an immune boost without the added sugar.

A number of the recipes that follow call for this base. The watermelon in the Watermelon Elderberry Slushie (page 127) and banana in banana "nice" cream (page 129), for example, are already so sweet, you wouldn't want to add sweetened syrup. **Makes approx. ⅔ cup**

½ cup dried elderberries (or 1 cup fresh)
2 cups filtered water

In a small saucepan, simmer berries and water, covered, over low heat for 30 minutes.

Turn off heat and allow to steep for at least an hour.

Strain and bottle, or use as your base for syrup or gummies.

Notes:
- The berries can be simmered again to make a weaker brew that you can drink as a tea. After you've drained the first batch, cover with a couple of inches of water and simmer another 20 minutes. You'll be surprised how dark and rich the liquid gets! You can drink this straight if you like. I sometimes get a third batch of still weaker tea after straining again. Though it's likely less medicinally powerful, it tastes good and is still a nice fruity herbal tea, if not what I'd turn to for battling flu.
- Elderberry base keeps in the refrigerator for about 5 days and takes on an unpleasant flavor after that. Freeze what you won't use well before then. You can put your concentrate in ice cube trays and defrost or just pop in freshly boiled water.
- If you're cooking up a batch for an acute cold or flu, you could try simmering the berries in coconut water, which will add some additional electrolytes. You can also add other herbs for additional benefits, like warming ginger or a bit of cinnamon. Find more ideas for herbs to consider on pages 46–50.

Simple Elderberry Syrup

Elderberry syrup involves a little more work than steeped tea, but not much, and simmering over low heat extracts more of the compounds we're after when we're fighting colds and flu. The honey has additional medicinal properties and acts as a preservative. This unspiced version may be used in gummies and other recipes, or you can try adding cinnamon, cloves, ginger, or other warming herbs included in Ultra Elderberry Syrup on page 104. **Makes about 1 cup**

½ cup dried elderberries
2 cups filtered water
⅓–½ cup raw honey

In a small saucepan, simmer berries in water over low heat for 30 minutes.

Allow to steep for at least an hour.

When cooled to almost room temperature, strain thoroughly, reserving berries.

Measure the liquid and add half as much honey. (If you have ⅔ cup liquid, add ⅓ cup honey). Stir in honey until fully incorporated.

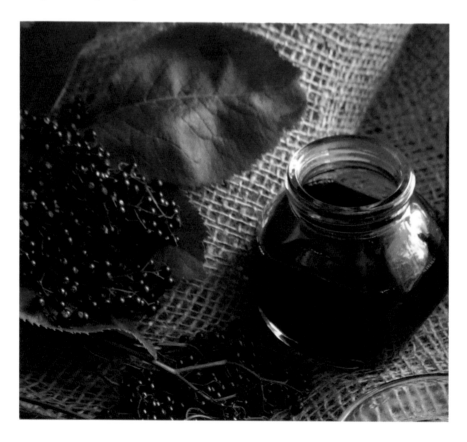

Notes:

- Berries can be simmered again to make a weaker brew that you can drink as a tea.
- For a stronger, thicker syrup, either use only 1½ cups of water or simmer longer to further reduce liquid before straining and adding honey.
- To make syrup from fresh berries: Freeze berries, then heat in a pot over very low heat with a very small amount of water to release the juice. Strain solids and measure, adding half as much honey as you have liquid. Because the berries don't cook long, the resulting liquid will be more of a juice and may not keep as long.
- Syrup made with cloves and cinnamon is reminiscent of mulled cider, which adds flavor you may not want in recipes like berry smoothies and rhubarb leather, so a simple syrup or base is called for in those recipes. But experiment and see what you like.
- This syrup is meant to be stored in the refrigerator and used within a few months. In the days before refrigeration, alcohol would be added as a preservative. If you would like to add alcohol, brandy is a common choice. You can add 1 part brandy to 4 parts syrup, or about 1 cup brandy to 1 quart syrup. Doubling the honey will also extend the shelf life, but it will make an extremely sweet syrup. You can also use water bath canning if you would like to preserve jars of syrup for longer, though the high heat may compromise the medicinal value of your syrup.
- Don't give honey to babies under one year of age. Substitute maple syrup or brown rice syrup if you plan to give to infants.
- Syrup can be used medicinally, taking a preventative spoonful daily or a spoonful a few times daily at the first sign of illness. It's also delicious as a pancake or ice cream topping, or swirled into yogurt or oatmeal.
- Some people make elderberry syrup in a pressure cooker or slow cooker. I have reservations about both. The high temperatures of the pressure cooker might compromise the beneficial compounds we're after, and the slow cooker might not get hot enough to address the compounds in *nigra* berries that give people trouble. Since neither makes a huge difference to the effort involved, it's probably best to stick with the traditional stovetop method.

Ultra Elderberry Syrup

If you really want to stoke your immune system, try simmering these immune-supporting, antiviral, anti-inflammatory herbs along with your elderberries (see more beginning on page 23). You can use all the additional ingredients, or pick and choose the ones you want. The amounts below are really suggestions, and you can develop your own favorite recipe by adjusting amounts to your liking. **Makes about 1 cup**

½ cup dried elderberries
2 cups water
1 tablespoon fresh ginger, peeled and chopped (or ¼ teaspoon dried)
½ teaspoon ground cinnamon
¼ teaspoon ground cloves
¼ cup rose hips
1 tablespoon astragalus
¼ teaspoon black pepper
⅓–½ cup raw honey

Place all ingredients except the honey in a pot, and simmer over low heat for 30 minutes. For a thicker syrup, continue to simmer over low heat until liquid is reduced by half. Strain thoroughly, squeezing solids in strainer to get out as much liquid as possible.

Measure the liquid and add half as much honey. If you have 1 cup liquid, add ½ cup honey. Stir in honey till fully incorporated.

Notes:
- Keep in an airtight container in the refrigerator for up to 3 months. This spiced syrup is delicious by the spoonful or stirred into hot water for a spicy, sweet tea.
- I prefer things less sweet, so I usually make this recipe with a 1:3 or 1:4 honey to elderberry ratio and use it more quickly than a syrup preserved with more sweetener.
- For a stronger, thicker syrup, either use only 1½ cups of water or simmer longer to further reduce liquid before straining and adding honey.

Elderberry-Infused Maple Sap

Ben Doherty, Open Hands Farm

I'm always especially drawn to recipes that make the most of natural abundance. Ben Doherty, one of the wonderful farmers who run the CSA we belong to, invented this ingenious way to sweeten their elderberry concoctions with nothing more than the sap running from a tree behind their house in late winter. I love that this recipe not only uses a thoroughly unprocessed form of sugar to sweeten elderberries, but if you have a mystical belief in the power of plant medicine, the sap running from a tree as winter changes to spring would seem especially useful for bracing against late-season colds. **Makes 1 quart**

2 quarts maple sap
¾ cup dried elderberries (or 1½ cups frozen berries)

Place sap and elderberries in a pot and bring to a boil.

Reduce to a simmer and cook until liquid is reduced by half.

Strain out berries, squeezing out all the liquid.

Store infused sap in the refrigerator for a few days, or freeze in an ice cube tray and defrost as needed.

Notes:
- If you don't have sap on hand, simmering berries in your favorite juice is another way to enjoy a lightly sweetened elderberry drink. If using juice, you don't need to boil it down. Use 1 quart juice, simmer 30 minutes, and allow to steep before straining.

Immune Boost Spruce Tea

There is so much to love about spruce tea: Besides smelling like Christmas, spruce is readily available all year round, making it a gift to the forager in winter, when foraging options get quite limited. A good source of vitamin C, it also contains shikimic acid, the active ingredient in Tamiflu, and pairs well with elderflower. Pine needles work also, though they typically have a stronger flavor. As with all foraging, consult a good guide to make sure you know what type of tree you're harvesting from. **Makes approx. 1 cup**

Large handful spruce tips, roughly a loose-packed cup
Boiling filtered water, enough to cover spruce
3–4 teaspoons Ultra Elderberry Syrup (page 104) per cup spruce tea

Infuse your spruce in boiling water for at least 10 minutes. I've found some spruce gives up its flavor more readily than others, so if you're not getting much flavor from infusing, you can simmer briefly on the stovetop.

Add elderberry syrup to taste.

Elderberry Tincture

While tincture sounds like something you need a degree in herbalism to make, tincturing is simply soaking herbs in alcohol, vinegar, or glycerine to extract their compounds. Tinctures extract different compounds than the water used in syrup-making or tea, and herbalists generally consider them more powerful than water-based preparations. You may use glycerine if you'd prefer an alcohol-free preparation, but most herbalists don't consider it as effective a solvent.

There are different schools of thought on how best to make tincture. Some herbalists prefer fresh berries and others favor dried, and the proportions of berries to alcohol recommended vary widely. Here's one option, but feel free to experiment with others to see what you prefer. **Makes approx. 1½ cups**

1 cup fresh elderberries (or ½ cup dried)
80- or 100-proof alcohol, such as brandy or vodka (or glycerine if you prefer alcohol-free)

Place elderberries in sterile pint jar and add alcohol or glycerine, covering the berries completely with a couple of inches of liquid and leaving about 1 inch of headroom from the top. Steep 4 to 8 weeks, shaking gently every few days, before straining out solids.

Store in a jar or glass dropper bottle out of direct sun. Keeps up to 5 years if using alcohol.

Because tinctures extract medicinal compounds so effectively, you use only very small amounts. At the first sign of illness, take a drop or two (at the low end of recommended dosages) or 4 to 6 mls (at the higher end) every hour to help fight off viral infections. (See page 40 for more information.)

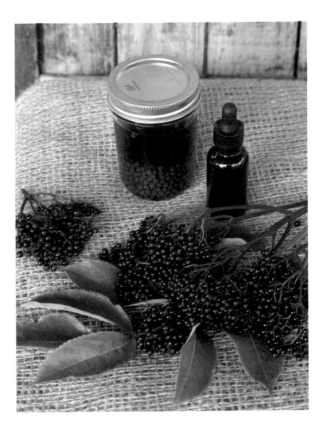

Elderberry-Infused Vinegar

This beautiful, fruity vinegar adds the goodness and flavor of elderberries to everything you use it in. I like to use apple cider vinegar for its extra probiotics, but other vinegars work also. Try in dressings and marinades, or combine with water and honey for a flavorful drink called a shrub. Or add to honey for an instant medicinal oxymel (page 111). **Makes approx. 1½ cups**

1 cup fresh elderberries (or ¼ cup dried)
Apple cider vinegar, red wine vinegar, or balsamic vinegar

Put elderberries in a pint jar and cover with vinegar of choice, leaving about 1 inch of headroom above the berries. Fruit may be mashed to encourage better extraction.

Cover with a plastic lid or place parchment paper or plastic film between the jar and metal lid.

Shake the jar to mix, and allow to steep in a cool, dark place such as a cupboard for 2 to 4 weeks, shaking every few days.

Strain and bottle.

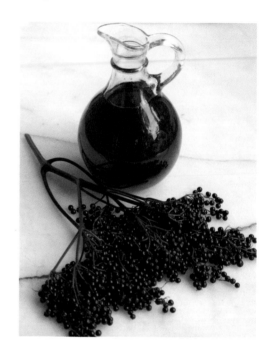

Note:
If using dried elderberries, flavors may extract better if the vinegar is hot or you simmer the berries for 10 minutes.

Elderflower-Infused Vinegar

This simple vinegar was a European kitchen staple for centuries and is a snap to make yourself. While the flavor is best with a neutral vinegar like white wine, you could also try apple cider vinegar. **Makes approx. 2 cups**

Several fresh elderflower heads (or about 1 cup dry)
2 cups white wine vinegar, or other vinegar of choice

Fill a sterile pint jar ⅔ full with fresh elderflowers or ½ full with dried elderflowers and cover completely with vinegar, leaving about 1 inch of headroom from the top. Use a plastic cap or place parchment paper or plastic film between the vinegar and metal lid. Steep 4 to 6 weeks, shaking gently every few days, before straining out solids.

While the main purpose of this vinegar is flavoring food, you can also use it medicinally, adding it to your Elderberry Switchel (page 159) or a vinaigrette any time you're dealing with respiratory symptoms.

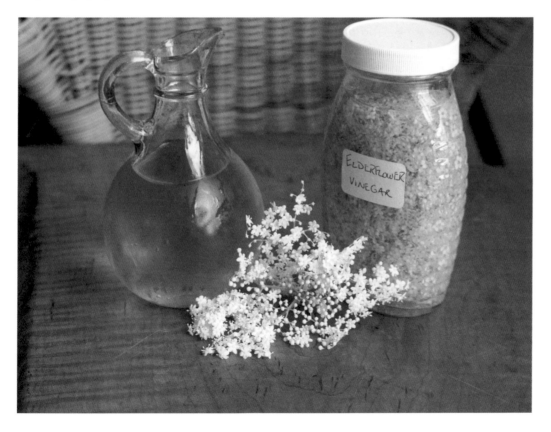

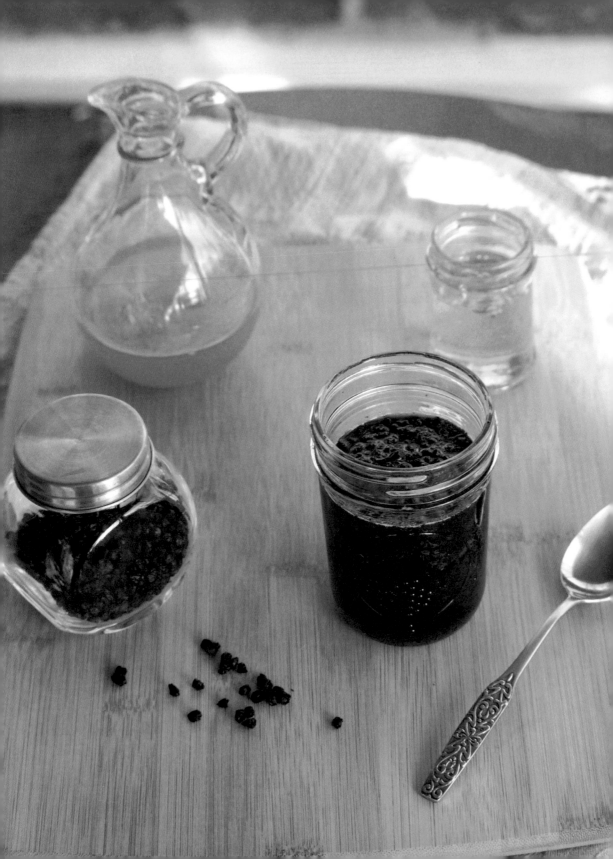

Elderberry Oxymel

This classic way to take medicine combines vinegar and honey with elderberries for a simple preventative syrup that's more shelf stable than elderberry syrup. You can vary the proportions of vinegar to honey to suit your tastes. This one isn't very sweet, but is somewhat reminiscent of balsamic vinegar. **Makes approx. 2 cups**

½ cup dried elderberries
1 cup apple cider vinegar
1 cup raw honey

Put elderberries in a pint jar with vinegar and honey, leaving about ½-inch headroom above the berries. Stir well.

Cover with a plastic lid or place parchment paper or plastic film between the jar and metal lid.

Store in a cool, dry place for 4 weeks, shaking every few days. Strain and bottle.

Elderflower Tincture

Like elderberry tincture, elderflower tincture is a simple recipe involving nothing more than elderflowers, vodka (or glycerine for alcohol-free), and time. **Makes approx. 1½ cups**

Several fresh elderflower heads, destemmed (or about 1 cup dry)
80- or 100-proof alcohol like vodka (or glycerine if you prefer alcohol-free)

Fill a sterile pint jar ⅔ full with fresh elderflowers or ½ full with dried elderflowers and cover completely with alcohol or glycerine, leaving about 1 inch of headroom from the top. Steep 4 to 8 weeks, shaking gently every few days, before straining out solids.

Store in a jar or glass dropper bottle out of direct sun. Keeps up to 5 years if using alcohol.

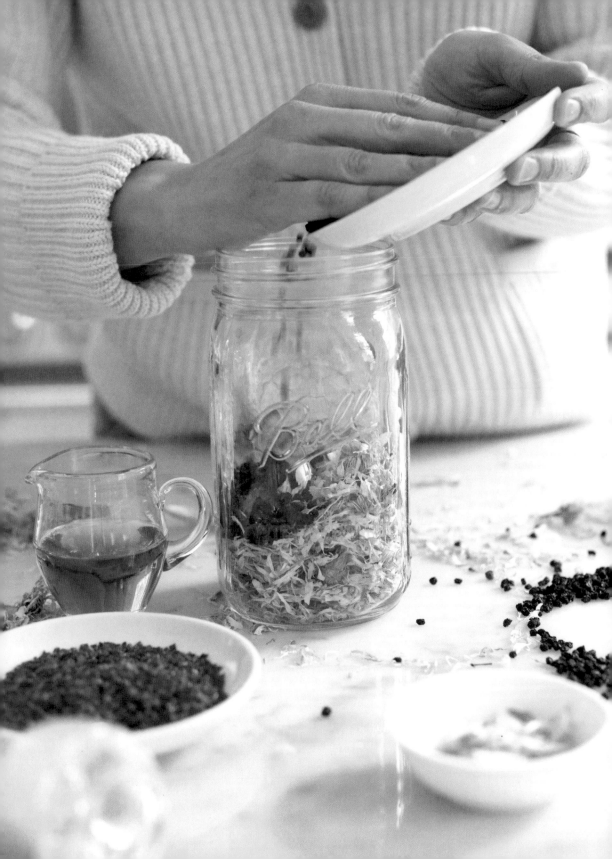

Elderberry Calendula Cold and Flu Elixir

Herbal Academy

This recipe is adapted from Kiva Rose Hardin's elderberry elixir and Kami McBride's cold and flu elixir, which use brandy to extract the plant constituents and honey to sweeten it up. The recipe is very versatile: you can use fresh or dried herbs and make additions or substitutions based on your own preferences. **Makes 2–3 cups**

1 cup fresh calendula flowers (or ⅔ cup dried)
⅔ cup dried elderberries
½ cup fresh elderflowers (or ⅓ cup dried)
½ cup fresh rose hips (or ⅓ cup dried)
2 tablespoons fresh orange peel (or 1 tablespoon dried)
1 tablespoon fresh ginger (or 1 teaspoon dried)
Brandy
Honey

Add herbs to a clean, sterilized quart jar.

Add brandy, pouring until herbs are covered by 1 to 2 inches of brandy and the jar is approximately ¾ full.

Add honey, leaving 1 inch of space at the top of the jar.

Poke a chopstick into jar to release any trapped air bubbles and ensure brandy and honey are coating herbs.

Put a cap on and label your jar with ingredients and date.

Let steep for 4 to 6 weeks in a cool, dark place, shaking daily.

Filter elixir by pouring through a fine mesh filter or several layers of cheesecloth over a bowl or wide-mouth jar. Press the plant material to squeeze out every last drop of elixir.

Compost the herbs, then cap and label the elixir.

Take 2–3 teaspoons elixir every 2–3 hours at the first sign of cold or flu. It may also be used as a preventative 2–3 times per day when a bug is going around.

Get-Well-Quick Elderberry Popsicle

This frozen treat is perfect for beating back colds and soothing sore throats with a winning combination of elderberry, elderflower, honey, and herbs from your Ultra Elderberry Syrup (page 104). You can also add elderberry syrup to any of your favorite juices and freeze. **Makes 1 popsicle**

For each popsicle:

¼ cup pomegranate, mango, or favorite juice blend

2 teaspoons Elderberry Base (page 101) or Syrup (page 102)

2 teaspoons Elderflower Infusion (page 98) or Syrup (page 123)

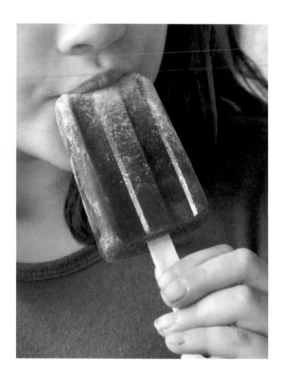

Combine ingredients, stir well, and taste. Add more syrup if needed.

Pour into popsicle molds.

Freeze 3 to 4 hours until frozen.

Note:
- If you'd like something less sweet, use elderflower infusion and elderberry base. Syrups will add a lot of sweetness if you use both.

Immune-Boosting Sore Throat Lollipops

Chrystal Johnson, Happy Mothering

These elderberry lollipops (or suckers, depending on the part of the country you're from) are a wonderful way to soothe sore throats, especially in kids too young for throat lozenges. Honey is excellent for soothing coughs and sore throats, and the elderberries, rose hips, cinnamon, and echinacea provide extra immune support. **Makes 12 pops**

2 tablespoons elderberries
2 tablespoons rose hips
2 tablespoons echinacea
1 cinnamon stick
2 cups filtered water
1½ cups organic honey
Slippery elm bark powder or vitamin C powder
    for dusting

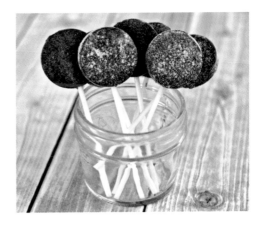

Add elderberries, rose hips, echinacea, and cinnamon stick to 2 cups of water and bring to a boil. Reduce heat to low and simmer 5 to 10 minutes. Cover the pan, remove from heat, and allow it to sit undisturbed for 30 minutes to allow the herbs to infuse.

Strain the herbs, then combine 1 cup of the herbal infusion with 1½ cups of honey in a medium-sized saucepan. Set the extra liquid aside. If you combine it with some raw honey, you'll have a delicious elderberry tea.

Heat the infusion and honey over medium heat until the temperature of the mixture reaches 300°F, approximately 30 minutes. You can test to see if it's done by putting a drop of the mixture into a glass of ice water. If it immediately hardens, it's done.

Immediately remove the pan from the heat. Stir until the bubbles dissipate.

Pour the mixture into your molds and insert sticks (or use a small silicone mold if you prefer to make lozenges). Do this quickly before the mixture hardens in the pan.

Allow the lollipops to cool completely.

Once they're cool, coat each side in slippery elm bark for extra throat soothing or vitamin C powder for extra immune boosting. The powder also helps keep them from sticking together.

Storing these in the fridge will keep them firm, and they'll also be less likely to stick together.

Peppermint Elderberry Cough Drops

Anna Merhalski, Salt in My Coffee

These soothing cough drops are sweetened with honey and are packed with the immune-boosting power of elderberries. Peppermint is not only a good flavor complement to elderberry, but also has natural decongestive properties to soothe a cough and dispel congestion. **Makes 48 small drops**

4 ounces dried elderberries, or 8 ounces fresh elderberries
½ cup dried peppermint leaves
2 cups water
1 cup honey

Add elderberries, peppermint, and water to a small saucepan. Bring to a gentle boil and simmer for 10 minutes. Berries will lose much of their color, and the liquid will look like grape juice.

Strain off the liquid, discarding the berries and mint leaves. Return strained liquid to the pan and add honey.

Stirring very frequently, simmer gently until the mixture reaches the "hard crack" stage, about 300°F on a candy thermometer. Drip a little drop from a spoon into a jar of ice water. When the drip turns into a very hard little ball (like a cough drop!), the mixture is ready.

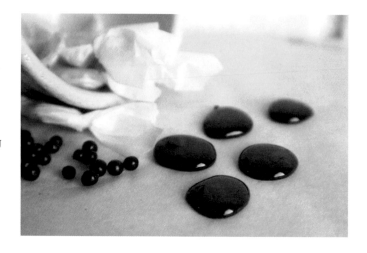

Pour hot mixture by teaspoonfuls onto parchment-lined cookie sheet, taking care that the drops don't touch each other.

When the cough drops are fully cooled, roll them up individually in squares of parchment paper.

Store in an airtight container in a cool, dry location.

PART II:
ELDERBERRY AND ELDERFLOWER DESSERTS, TREATS & MORE

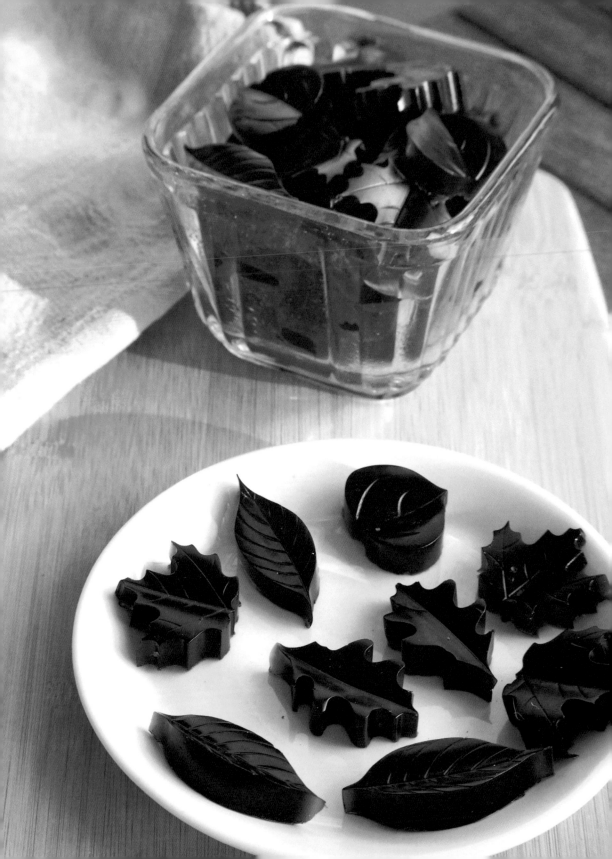

Elderberry Gummies

Elderberry gummies are a fun and yummy way to fight off illness, tasting much more like a treat than medicine. We use fun-shaped silicone molds that appeal to kids, but you can also pour the liquid into a glass baking pan and cut it into cubes if you'd rather.

The nourishing gelatin is a good way to get in some nutrition and is reportedly good for gut health, which in turn supports the immune system. We use juice to temper the strong flavor of the elderberry, but you can make it with nothing but elderberry syrup as well. **Makes about 30 gummies**

3 tablespoons grass-fed gelatin
½ cup room-temperature fruit juice (dark pomegranate and cherry blends work especially well, but mango and apple are also good)
½ cup Simple Elderberry Syrup (page 102)

Start by getting your molds ready. Silicone molds are floppy, so place them on a plate or cookie sheet to help you get them to the fridge without spilling.

Sprinkle gelatin over your juice and allow to sit a few minutes to hydrate.

If you've just made syrup, allow it to cool. If your syrup is cold, warm it in a pot on the stove over low heat. You want it hot, but not boiling.

Add gelatin and juice mixture to syrup, whisking until completely dissolved. You can heat it briefly while you do this if the gelatin isn't dissolving.

When the gelatin has completely dissolved, allow to cool about 10 minutes before pouring into prepared molds.

Use a measuring cup to pour into molds; for very small molds, a dropper may work better.

Refrigerate until set, about an hour.

Pop gummies out of molds and place in airtight container. Keeps in the refrigerator for up to 5 days.

Notes:
- We prefer Simple Elderberry Syrup (page 102) or Elderberry Base (page 101) to make gummies, but you can simmer any additional herbs you like with the berries before making gummies or use the Ultra Elderberry Syrup (page 104) for a spiced gummy. Using elderflower tea or infusion in place of some of the juice is another option.
- If you want to make gummies with only elderberry syrup, use 3 tablespoons of gelatin per cup of liquid.
- For a vegan gummy, try 4½ teaspoons of agar powder in place of the gelatin.

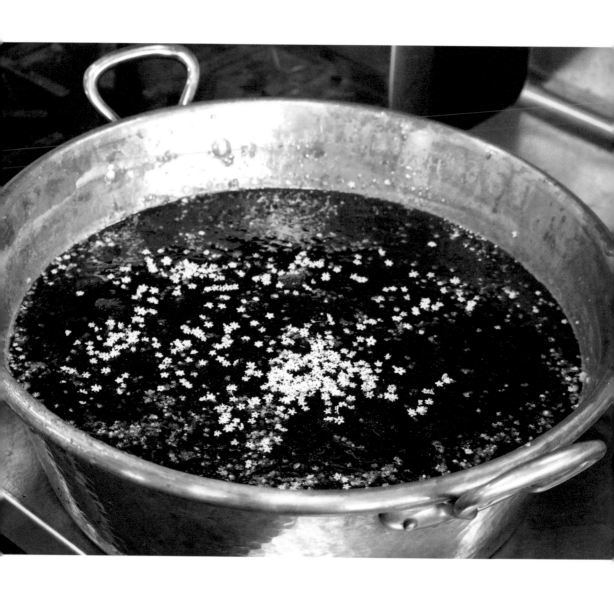

Strawberry Elderflower Jam

Heidi Skoog, Serious Jam

This decadent jam bursts with the flavor of fresh-picked spring fruits and flowers. A top seller at Serious Jam in Saint Paul, Minnesota, it makes a beautiful gift if you don't eat it all yourself! **Makes about 8 (8-ounce) jars**

5 pounds hulled strawberries
3 pounds sugar
1–2 ounces fresh lemon juice
3–5 heads elderflower blossoms

Place berries in a large bowl and layer in the sugar and lemon juice. Cover tightly and let berries macerate in the refrigerator for 2 to 5 days. Stir once a day to dissolve sugar.

When you're ready to make your jam, gather fresh elderflowers on a dry morning. Remove the flowers from the stems, leaving just the blossoms.

Set aside in the refrigerator, placing a slightly damp paper towel over the top of them until ready to use.

Remove the berry mixture from the refrigerator and stir well to dissolve any undissolved sugar. Taste the liquid and adjust with lemon juice. It should taste like strawberries first, not sugar. If it doesn't, add in a bit more lemon juice until it tastes of bright fruit.

Place a small plate or several spoons in the freezer. You will use them to check jam for set later on.

Transfer berry mixture to a preserving pan or wide stockpot and gently bring to a boil, stirring frequently to dissolve any remaining undissolved sugar.

Continue cooking until it comes to a rolling boil, then reduce heat slightly, continuing to cook until mixture becomes thick and dark, around 219°F. It will foam up in the beginning, so pay attention and adjust heat and stir to avoid boiling over. When it looks finished, remove from heat and test for set by placing a small amount of jam on your plate or a spoon from freezer. Let cool for a minute and tilt the spoon or plate to see how fast the jam runs off. It should be slow moving and jam-like. If it is too liquid, bring it back to a boil for another 30 seconds or so and test again.

When satisfied with the set, add in the elderflower blossoms. Taste and adjust as needed. If it is too sweet, add in a bit more lemon juice to balance it out.

Pour into warm, clean, sterilized jars and seal. Store in the refrigerator when cool. Alternatively, you can "water-bath process" the jam for 10 minutes. Jam will be shelf stable for a year, but tastes best if eaten within 8 months.

Elderberry Raspberry Chia Jam

Chia jam is a quick and easy way to make a low-sugar jam with minimal fuss. Chia works as a thickener and adds some extra nutrition. This recipe can be made in small amounts when you have just a couple of heads of berries, or multiplied if you want to make more.

Because elderberries are so seedy, this jam is also seedy. Just a heads-up for those who don't love seedy jams, or those sensitive to elderberry seeds. You can experiment with adding other berries, like strawberries or blackberries, as well. **Makes approx. 8 ounces**

1½ cups fresh elderberries
½ cup raspberries
½ teaspoon lemon juice
2 tablespoons chia seeds
2 tablespoons honey

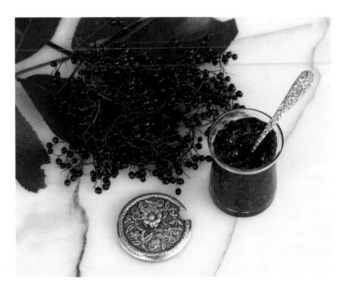

Put berries in a saucepan and cook over very low heat, stirring frequently and mashing with a fork, spoon, or potato masher.

When the fruit is well heated and begins to bubble, add the lemon juice and chia seeds and stir to combine.

Remove from heat and add honey, mixing well.

Let the jam cool and set up, then jar and refrigerate.

Keeps about 1 week in the refrigerator.

Elderflower Syrup

A simple syrup made with nothing more than flowers, water, and sugar, elderflower syrup makes a decadent flavoring you can add to cake frosting, drinks, or use as a topping for things like pancakes and yogurt. (Several recipes below call for it.) The flavor rather than the medicinal properties is the point here—the sugar makes it hard to call this a health food! So enjoy it as a delightful flavoring that captures the scent of summer rather than turning to it when you have a cold. **Makes approx. 2½ cups**

1 cup elderflowers, stems removed
½ organic lemon, sliced into rounds
2 cups filtered water
1 cup sugar
1½ teaspoons fresh lemon juice

Place flowers and lemon slices in a bowl or jar.

Heat water and sugar in a saucepan until sugar dissolves. Do not allow to boil.

Add lemon juice and stir.

Allow the sugar syrup to cool.

Pour warm sugar syrup over flowers and lemon, and cover. Allow to steep in the refrigerator for 1 to 4 days, stirring daily.

Use a fine sieve to strain out solids, and transfer to an airtight container.

> **Notes:**
> - Many elderflower syrup-makers save time by steeping whole umbels upside down in the sugar water. I prefer to remove as much stem as possible to keep the less desirable compounds and flavors out, but the choice is yours.
> - Syrup will keep in the refrigerator for up to a month. Freeze in ice-cube trays to preserve longer. (A cube in a tall glass of seltzer makes an absolutely delicious homemade soda.)

Immune-Boosting
Triple Berry Smoothie

When there's a bug going around and you want to give your immune system a little extra support, try the one-two punch of elderberries and probiotic-rich yogurt. Blend up with some vitamin C–filled frozen raspberries, strawberries, and broccoli, plus magnesium-rich chia seeds, and you have a tangy treat that gives your body the nutrients it needs to keep you healthy. **Makes 2 servings**

1 cup yogurt
1 tablespoon chia seeds
1 cup frozen strawberries and raspberries, any proportion
¼ cup Simple Elderberry Syrup (page 102)
2 tablespoons frozen broccoli or spinach

Put yogurt and chia in a blender and blend to allow chia to absorb moisture. Add remaining ingredients and blend well. Serve immediately for a slightly frozen treat, or put in the refrigerator for more of a blended drink.

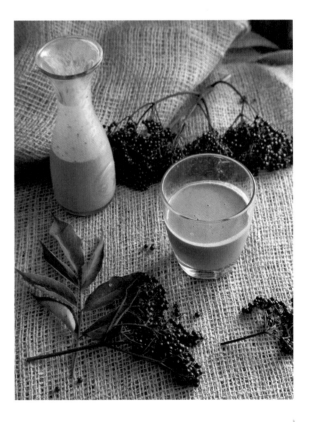

Elderberry Lemonade Pops

This slightly healthier twist on the popsicle has a delicious tart sweetness that's perfect for cooling off on a hot day. Elderberry and lemon combine beautifully in this frozen treat, and it's a snap to put together. **Makes 4 popsicles**

1 cup lemonade (homemade or purchased)
2 tablespoons elderberry base

Combine lemonade and elderberry base.

Pour into popsicle molds and freeze for 3 to 4 hours.

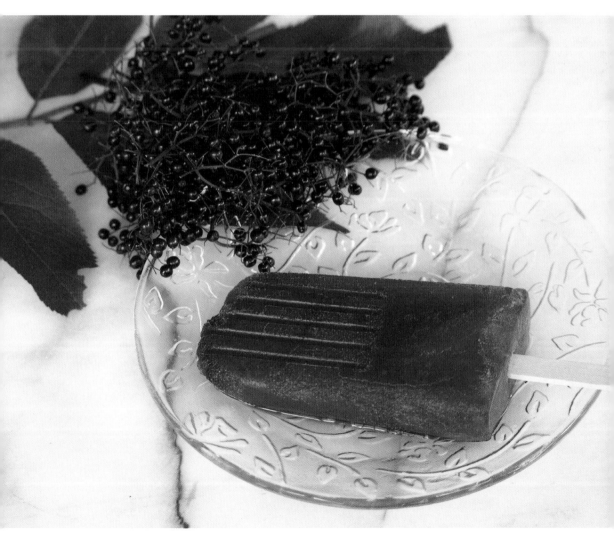

Blueberry-Elderberry Frozen Yogurt Pops

These beautiful purple popsicles are both delicious and loaded with healthy nutrients. Protein, probiotics, polyphenols, and intense flavor—who could ask for anything more in a cool summer treat? Because syrups can vary so widely in concentration, I recommend tasting your yogurt mixture and adding more elderberry syrup if you'd like a stronger flavor. **Makes 6 to 8 popsicles**

1 cup blueberries
1 cup yogurt
3-4 tablespoons Simple Elderberry Syrup (page 102)

Add all ingredients to your blender and blend until smooth.

Pour into popsicle molds and freeze for 3 to 4 hours or until frozen.

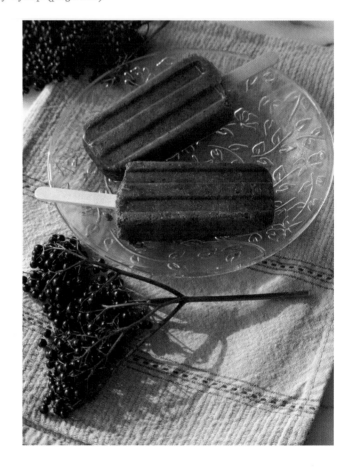

Watermelon Elderberry Slushie

Frozen watermelon and elderberry blends into a refreshing, healthy, sugar-free slushie. Serve to kids in place of chemically-flavored and colored options, or as a light dessert in a bowl with a spoon. **Makes 1 to 2 servings**

2½ cups seedless watermelon, cubed
2 tablespoons Elderberry Base (page 101)

Place cubed watermelon in the freezer for 3 to 4 hours or until frozen. Put frozen watermelon in a blender with elderberry base and blend on high until smooth. Serve immediately in a bowl with a spoon for something like a soft sorbet, or in a glass with a straw.

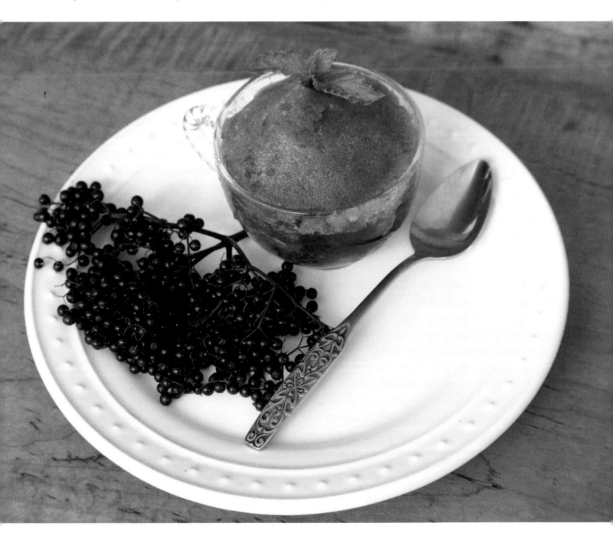

Melon Elderflower "Sorbet"

This easy sorbet capitalizes on the natural sweetness of melon and the delicate flavor of elderflower. Make it with elderflower liqueur instead of syrup for a delicious grown-up dessert or frozen drink. Because melons and elder products vary so much in flavor and sweetness, use the amounts below as a guideline and adjust according to taste. **Makes 4 servings**

4 cups cubed watermelon or honeydew, seeds removed
5 tablespoons Elderflower Syrup (page 123), or 3 tablespoons Elderflower Liqueur (page 164)

Put cubed watermelon in the freezer for 3 to 4 hours or until frozen.

Place in a blender with syrup or liqueur and blend on high until smooth. Add more syrup if desired.

Serve immediately in a bowl with a spoon as a soft sorbet. It melts quickly, so you can also serve it in a glass with a straw as a frozen drink.

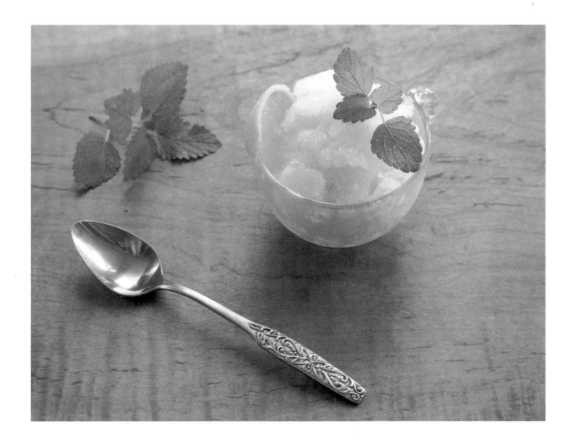

Blueberry, Peach & Elderberry "Nice" Cream

This vegan dessert uses frozen bananas that transform into a creamy non-dairy soft-serve ice cream that pairs well with berry and peach flavors. This is a healthy but decadent dessert loaded with nutrients, and a delicious way to get your daily dose of elderberry! **Makes 4 servings**

2 cups sliced bananas, frozen until solid
3 tablespoons Elderberry Base (page 101)
Squeeze of fresh lemon
Splash of almond milk or other milk of choice
2 cups frozen blueberries
1 cup frozen peach or nectarine pieces

Place bananas, base, lemon juice, and milk in blender and pulse to combine.

Add half the blueberries and peach and blend until ingredients start to get smooth.

Add the rest of the frozen fruit and blend until creamy, scraping down the sides as needed.

Best eaten immediately, as the texture won't be as creamy after it refreezes.

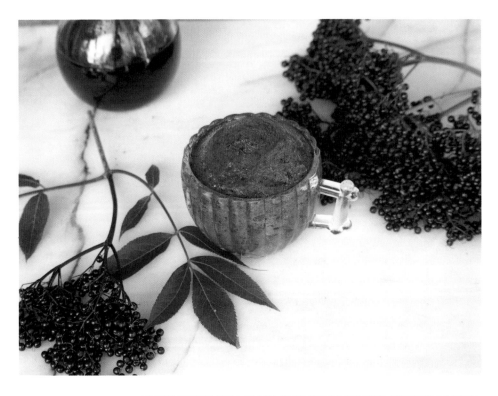

Elderflower and Lemon Ice Cream in an Elderflower Ice Bowl

Belvoir Farms

As if homemade ice cream flavored with elderflowers wasn't impressive enough, this recipe serves it up in a beautiful ice bowl studded with lovely elder blossoms. **Makes about 1½ pints**

6 eggs, yolks and whites separated
4 ounces caster sugar
¾ cup Belvoir Elderflower Cordial or homemade Elderflower Syrup (page 123)
2 tablespoons grated lemon peel
20 ounces double cream
Optional extra: Broken up caramelized nut brittle

For the ice cream:
Beat egg whites until stiff, either in a stand mixer or by hand—this should take a few minutes. Then gradually beat in sugar.

In another medium-sized bowl, beat egg yolks until they begin to thicken, then beat in elderflower syrup and lemon peel.

Whip cream briefly with a whisk and then fold into egg yolk mixture and egg whites.

Place in a freezer container overnight to freeze. There is no need to re-whip.

For the ice bowl:
You need one freezable bowl which will fit inside another larger bowl, some slices of lemon, a collection of elderflower sprigs and leaves, and some honey.

Brush insides of the bigger bowl with honey to help stick on the flowers.

Place a few slices of lemon on the base of the larger bowl and place smaller bowl on top. Weight smaller bowl with a bag of frozen peas.

Place leaves, flower heads, and remaining lemon slices in the gap between the bowls. Add water to fill the gap completely. Freeze for 30 minutes until water begins to freeze.

Periodically push down the flowers, leaves, and lemons into the freezing water, adding more water as necessary to fill the gap between the bowls.

Freeze for 24 hours.

Remove frozen bowls from freezer and remove bag of peas. Pour warm water into small bowl to loosen it from larger bowl.

Dip large bowl in warm water and then tip ice bowl out. Return to freezer until ready to use.

Take ice cream out of freezer to slightly soften.

At point of service, place ice bowl on a plate and fill with frozen ice cream.

Once placed in individual bowls, caramelized nut brittle may be sprinkled on top.

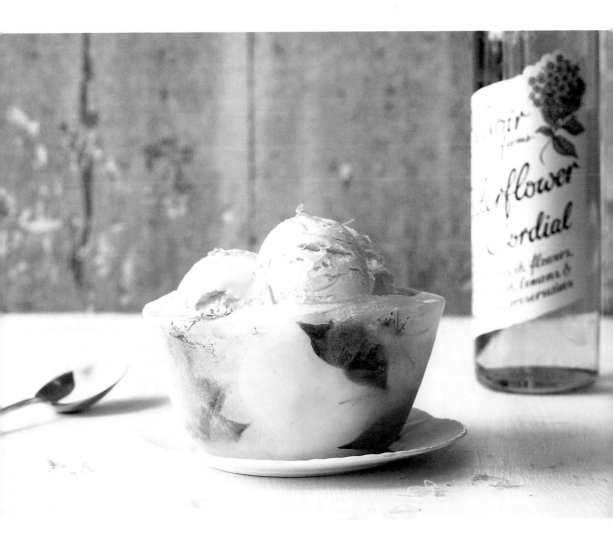

Chocolate Syrup with Elderberries and Rose Hips

Rosalee de la Forêt

This syrup is antioxidant-rich, combining the health benefits of cocoa with the beneficial medicine of elderberries and nutrient-rich rose hips. Cinnamon is known for many health benefits, including its ability to regulate blood sugar and body temperature and relieve digestive complaints, arthritic pain, and menstrual cramping. Nutmeg can promote digestion and sexual health, and act as a sedative. When you take your first bite of this delicacy, don't pay any attention to the fact that it can support your heart health, boost your immune system, and prevent sickness. Just enjoy that incredible flavor. **Makes approx. 1½ cups**

½ cup elderberries
½ cup rose hips
2 cups water
2 tablespoons 100% cocoa powder
1 teaspoon cinnamon
Pinch freshly grated nutmeg
Honey, to taste

Simmer the elderberries and rose hips in 2 cups of water for 20 minutes. Strain well.

Whisk in the cocoa powder, cinnamon, and nutmeg. Add honey to taste while the mixture is still warm. Mix well.

This syrup can be drizzled on ice cream, bananas, or enjoyed on pancakes.

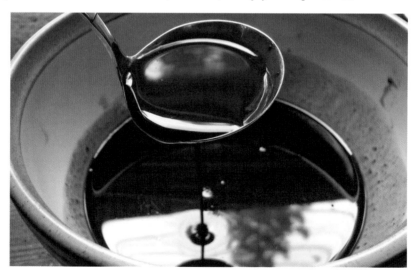

Zucchini Elderflower Muffins

Elderflowers reach their peak as the first zucchinis start trickling in, and the delicate flowers on this muffin make it something special. I like to keep muffins on the healthy side so they can be breakfast or a snack rather than dessert, so this recipe features whole grains, healthy fat, and less sugar than many. The flavor of the flowers is very subtle, and if you choose to add lemon zest—which is delicious!—it may overpower the elderflower. Using fresh-picked elderflowers with plenty of pollen for both the syrup and the muffin will help make the flavor more pronounced. **Makes 12 muffins**

2 cups white whole wheat flour
½ cup coconut sugar
1 tablespoon baking powder
½ teaspoon salt
2 large eggs
¾ cup milk
2 tablespoons Elderflower Syrup
  (page 123)
⅓ cup melted coconut oil
1 cup zucchini, shredded and well-
  drained (reserve the juice for
  soup)
¾ cup fresh elderflower blossoms,
  plus extra for sprinkling on top of
  batter
1 teaspoon lemon zest (optional)

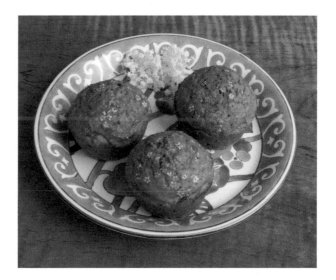

Preheat oven to 350°F.

In a large bowl, combine dry ingredients and mix well.

In a separate bowl, beat the eggs with milk and elderflower syrup. Add oil and mix.

Fold wet ingredients into the dry ingredients, along with the zucchini, elderflower blossoms, and zest, if using. Mix till just combined.

Spoon into muffin tin. Add extra flowers on top, making sure they're incorporated into the batter.

Bake about 20 minutes and check for doneness by inserting a cake tester or toothpick, which will come out clean when fully cooked.

Elderberry Raspberry Baked Oatmeal

A major step up from regular oatmeal and packed with nutritious ingredients, baked oatmeal is sort of a cross between plain ol' oatmeal and an oat muffin. It has a heartier texture than a muffin, and more protein and other nutrients than a regular bowl of oatmeal. I love digging into something that feels a little indulgent but is still a pretty healthy way to start the day. I like to soak the oats overnight to break down phytates and make the nutrients more available. **Makes 6 servings**

3 cups rolled oats
1 tablespoon chia seeds
2 teaspoons flaxseed meal
½ cup plain yogurt
¾ cup milk of choice
½ cup applesauce
½ cup coconut sugar, honey, or maple syrup

2 teaspoons baking powder
¼ teaspoon salt
¼ cup oil or butter
1 teaspoon vanilla
4 medium eggs
2 cups fresh or frozen raspberries
1 cup fresh or frozen elderberries

The night before you want to bake your oatmeal, combine oats, chia, flax, yogurt, and milk in a large bowl and cover with a tea towel.

In the morning, preheat your oven to 350°F. To your bowl, add applesauce, sweetener, baking powder, salt, oil, vanilla, and eggs, and mix well to combine. Fold in berries.

Grease an 8x8-inch baking dish with butter or coconut oil, and transfer oatmeal mixture.

Bake for about 45 minutes, until top is golden and a knife comes out clean.

Cool before serving. Will keep in the refrigerator for up to 1 week.

Notes:

- The tartness of the raspberry sets off the rich-flavored elderberry nicely, but other berries would work as well. You could add in a half-cup of walnuts, pecans, or sliced almonds if you'd like to add extra depth and nutrition.
- I like the extra chewy texture of thick rolled oats, but any "old fashioned" rolled oats will work. Look for certified gluten-free rolled oats if you want to make this completely free of gluten, which sometimes contaminates oat crops.
- If you don't have fresh or frozen elderberries, you can rehydrate dry ones, but I generally find their texture a little off-putting, like raisins that got too dried out. To rehydrate dried elderberries, cover with boiling water and allow to sit overnight before putting in your oatmeal. You might drink the liquid as a tea.

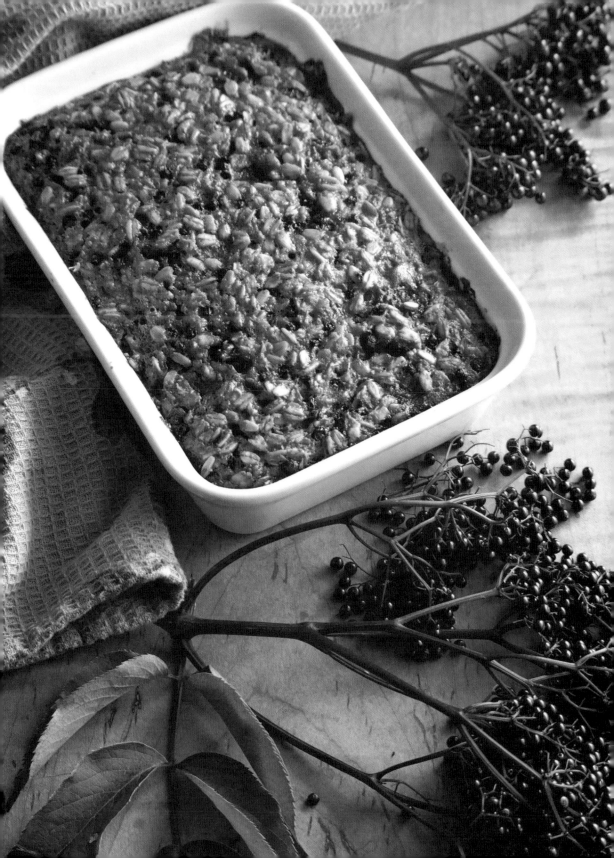

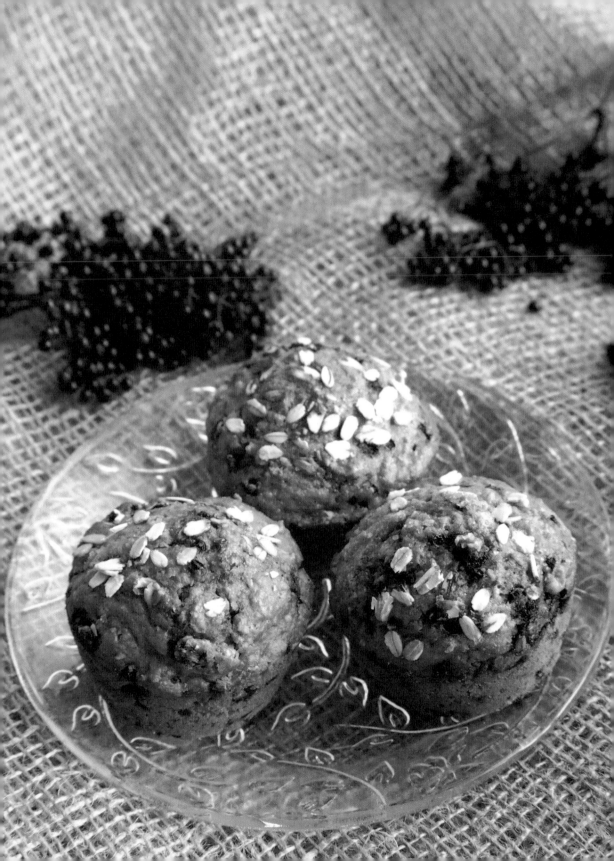

Foraged Berry Oat Muffins

Even if you don't have a chance to do much foraging, collecting a couple cups of berries over the course of the summer is totally doable. I nearly missed the black raspberry season, but I managed to grab a couple of handfuls and stow them in a container in the freezer. Then as the mulberries trickled in, I added them a few at a time. Come elderberry season, I was ready with enough mixed berries for these fun and hearty muffins. Use whatever combination of berries you get! Tart black or red raspberries are especially good, and you could also use blackberries, mulberries, blueberries, or whatever berries grow near you. **Makes 12 muffins**

1½ cups white whole wheat flour
½ cup quick oats
½ cup coconut sugar
1 tablespoon baking powder
½ teaspoon salt
2 large eggs, room temperature
½ cup milk, room temperature
⅓ cup lemon juice
¼ cup melted coconut oil or butter
2 cups mixed foraged berries
1 tablespoon grated lemon zest
1 teaspoon demerara sugar, optional

Preheat oven to 375°F.

Grease a muffin pan. In a bowl, combine the dry ingredients and mix well.

In a separate bowl, beat the eggs with milk and lemon juice. Add melted oil and mix.

Add dry ingredients and mix till just combined. Allow to sit a few minutes so oats can absorb moisture.

Fold in berries and lemon zest.

Spoon into muffin tin, and top with a sprinkle of sugar if desired.

Bake about 20 minutes, or until a toothpick or cake tester comes out clean.

Elderberry Rhubarb Fruit Leather

As treats go, you can't get much healthier than a fruit leather made with a vegetable and a "super" berry. If you don't mind the seediness, you could use fresh, frozen, or rehydrated elderberries in this recipe, but I think it works better with elderberry syrup (or base plus sweetener). Rhubarb and elderberry complement each other beautifully, though it can take a fair amount of sweetening when you use two tart ingredients. **Makes about 16 leather strips**

4 cups chopped rhubarb stalks (leaves are poisonous and should be discarded)
3 tablespoons Simple Elderberry Syrup (page 102)
Stevia, sugar, honey, or other sweetener to taste

Cut rhubarb into ½-inch pieces and place in a large pot. Cover with filtered water and bring almost to a boil, then turn off the heat. Let sit about an hour to allow the rhubarb to soften.

Scoop rhubarb with a slotted spoon into a blender or food processor.* Add elderberry syrup and blend. Taste, then add sugar, honey, stevia, or other sweetener if desired. The final leather will be sweeter than the sauce, so keep the sauce on the tart side. The sauce should be

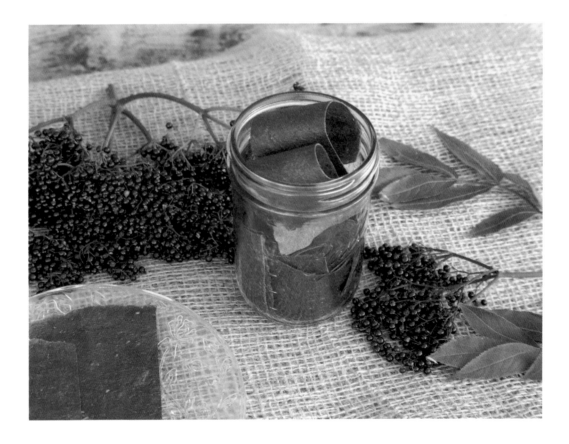

deliciously (rather than unpleasantly) tart and tastes great as a dessert or topping for yogurt or ice cream if you have a little left over.

*I recommend keeping the liquid. It's great on its own, added to lemonade, or with a splash of elderberry base. See Rhubarb Elderberry Cooler on page 157.

Dehydrator instructions:
Spray (or brush lightly) vegetable oil on the leather-making discs to keep the leather from sticking.

Spread sauce about ¼-inch thick, as evenly as possible. If you can see the white of the disc, your sauce is too thin.

Set the temperature to 130°F and let run for about 4 hours. Check if it's dried into leather but still pliable; allow to dehydrate further if some parts are still sauce rather than leather.

Oven instructions:
Line 2 cookie sheets with a silpat mat and oil lightly. Set your oven to the lowest temperature possible. Check after two hours and return to the oven if some of it is still sauce rather than leather.

Keep in an airtight container for up to a year, though I doubt you will have any left after a few weeks!

Notes:
- This recipe makes enough to fill two leather discs if you're using a dehydrator or about two baking trays if you're using an oven. One disc can get gobbled up pretty fast, so I often do an entire stockpot of rhubarb and make a huge batch of leather at once. You can double, triple, or quadruple the recipe to fill more dehydrator trays and use any remaining trays to dry other fruits.
- If you choose to use whole elderberries, note that since rhubarb is ready in late spring and elderberries don't come in till the end of summer, you'll need to freeze your rhubarb and save it till elderberry time, or use frozen or dried elderberries.

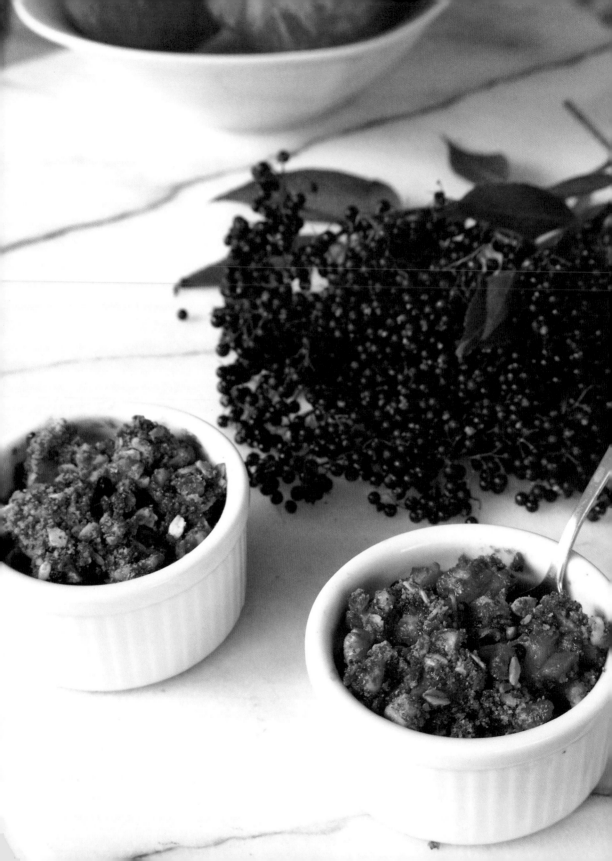

Elderberry Apple Crisp

The 1997 revised and updated Joy of Cooking *no longer included the elderberry recipes from prior editions, but there is a note recommending elderberries as the top fruit for adding "verve" to apple pies. This twist on a traditional apple crisp uses elderberry syrup and fresh elderberries to add color and flavor—maybe even verve?—to the apples. This crisp will taste best with larger, sweeter elderberries such as* cerulea *or Bob Gordon. If the only berries you can get are on the bland side, soaking them in the syrup helps improve their flavor.* **Makes 4 to 6 servings**

For the fruit base:
⅔ cup fresh or frozen elderberries
6 tablespoons Ultra Elderberry Syrup (page 104)
2 teaspoons lemon juice
4 cups sliced apples
2 teaspoons Ceylon cinnamon

For the crisp topping:
4 tablespoons butter (use coconut oil for vegan)
¾ cup brown or coconut sugar, loosely packed
½ cup white whole wheat flour (or flour of choice)
½ teaspoon Ceylon cinnamon
½ cup rolled oats (I use thick rolled oats)
½ cup walnuts (omit for nut allergies)

For the fruit base: Place berries, syrup, and lemon juice in a bowl and allow to soak for at least an hour, but preferably overnight.

Preheat oven to 350°F. Place apples in a greased 8x8-inch baking dish, add cinnamon, and toss to coat evenly. Sprinkle your soaked berry mixture on top, and gently combine, trying to keep all the berries from falling to the bottom of the dish.

For the topping: Put butter, brown sugar, flour, and cinnamon in a food processor and pulse 20 to 30 seconds, till it forms little balls.

Add oats and nuts, and pulse a few times to combine.

Crumble the topping over apples and bake until golden, about 45 minutes.

Note: If you have sweeter, more flavorful berries, try using only ¼ cup syrup.

Elderberry Tarts

Ashley Adamant, Practical Self Reliance

Elderberry tarts are delicious and surprisingly easy, and they work well with either fresh or dried elderberries. Just a few cups of elderberries and you're well on your way to a miniature version of old-fashioned elderberry pie. **Makes 6 to 8 tarts**

Crust:
2¼ cups flour
½ teaspoon salt
1 cup butter
4–6 tablespoons water, cold

Filling:
1 cup sugar
3–4 tablespoons cornstarch (or tapioca starch)
½ cup water (see note)
4 cups elderberries, rinsed and de-stemmed
2 tablespoons lemon juice

For the crust: Mix flour and salt (with a tablespoon of sugar, if desired) and then cut the butter into the flour mixture until crumbly.

Add water and bring the mixture together into a cohesive mass.

Divide into two pieces, cover each with plastic wrap, and refrigerate.

For the filling: Place the sugar, cornstarch, and water in a saucepan large enough to hold all the filling.

Bring the mixture to a boil, stirring to dissolve.

Add elderberries and lemon juice and cook another 2 to 3 minutes until heated through. Set aside to cool slightly while you prepare the crust.

Preheat oven to 425°F.

Remove one half of the crust from the refrigerator, roll it out, and use it to line tart pans.

Fill the crust with the elderberry pie filling, and then top with the second half of the crust (as a lattice top or solid top pie).

Seal the edges, and optionally, paint the top with milk or egg white for a golden crust. A sprinkle of sugar on top is also a nice decorative touch.

Bake for 30 minutes and then reduce the oven temperature to 350°F for an additional 20 to 30 minutes until the crust is browned and the filling bubbly.

Allow the pie to cool completely before cutting.

Notes:

- The recipe includes ½ cup water to dissolve the cornstarch and sugar for the filling, but elderberry juice (or elderberry tea made from dried elderberries) would be a more flavorful choice.
- Can be made with either fresh or dried elderberries. If using dried, rehydrate 2 cups dried fruit in 3 cups water overnight. Add the fruit (and remaining soaking water) to a saucepan and proceed with the recipe as if you'd used fresh elderberries.

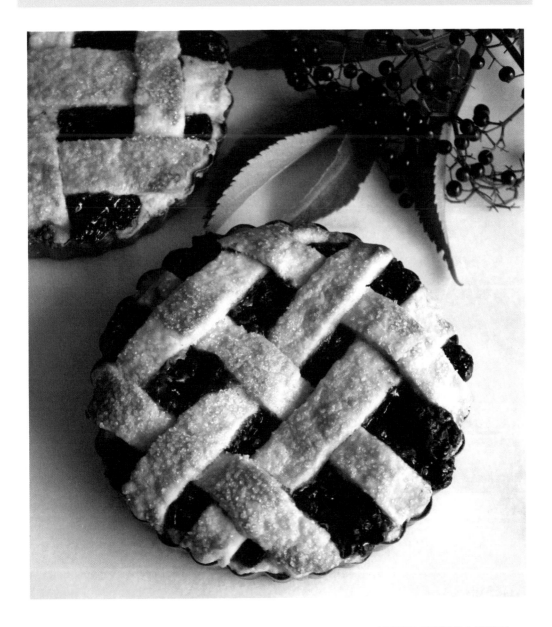

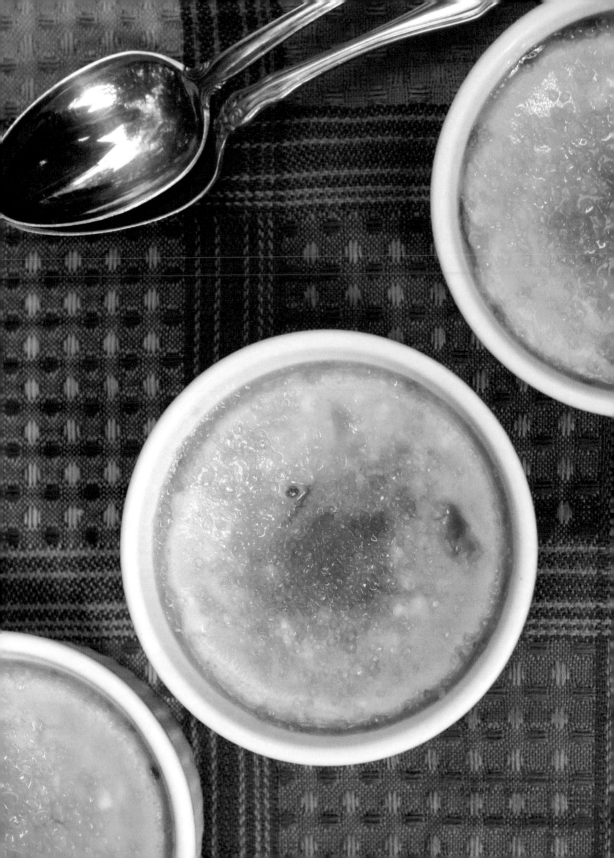

Elderflower Flan

Ann Lenhardt, Norm's Farms

Flan, an egg and cream-based dish, dates back all the way to the Roman empire. The dish made use of commonly available ingredients, and both savory and sweet versions of the recipe have been popular in cultures all around the world. Elderflower syrup works beautifully in this dessert, and using whole milk instead of cream saves a bit on the calories, too. **Makes 8 servings**

4 eggs
3 cups milk
¾ cup elderflower syrup

Preheat oven to 350°F.

Whip eggs in a bowl until lightly beaten.

Add milk and elderflower syrup, and gently beat until well combined.

Pour mixture into 8 half-cup ramekins.

Arrange ramekins in a baking dish. Pour enough water into baking dish to come halfway up the sides of the ramekins.

Place in preheated oven and bake 50 to 60 minutes until a knife inserted in the center of the custard comes out clean.

Remove ramekins from the baking dish and place in the fridge to cool for at least an hour.

Before serving, sprinkle turbinado sugar on the top of each flan.

Using a torch, melt the sugar to form a crispy top and serve.

Can be made one day ahead.

Pontack Sauce

Hunter, Angler, Gardener, Cook

I first heard of pontack when I read about it in the excellent book The River Cottage Preserves Handbook, *which is by one of Britain's master preservers, Pam Corbin. When I began researching this vinegary elderberry sauce, it seemed to be an ancient British recipe, dating back at least a few centuries. This sauce, which mellows with age—it can age for many years—is a spicy, zingy, fruity foil for simple meats, whether they were grilled or boiled or anything else.* **Makes 1 pint**

2 pounds fresh elderberries, destemmed (or 12 ounces dried)
4 cups cider vinegar
1 pound shallots, minced
10 allspice berries
1 teaspoon nutmeg
2 tablespoons cracked black peppercorns
1 teaspoon salt

Preheat your oven to 250°F. Put the elderberries into a covered casserole or other oven-proof dish with the vinegar and cook for 4 to 6 hours. Your house will smell like fruity vinegar during this time, which isn't such a bad thing.

Pour the cooked liquid through a strainer and into a large bowl. Let the cooked berries cool enough to handle. Then, with your clean hands, press as much juice as you can from the berries and into the bowl. You might need to do this in batches. Discard the spent berries.

Pour the sauce into a pot and add the remaining ingredients. Simmer gently for 25 minutes. Strain one more time to remove the spices.

Return it to the pot and bring it to a boil; let it boil for 5 minutes.

Meanwhile, get very clean mason jars or other sterile containers. This sauce is primarily vinegar, so you really don't have to worry too much about it going bad.

Pour the hot pontack into your containers and seal. Let cool and put in your pantry. Should last at least a year, and likely much longer.

Elderberry Chutney

Marion Harris Neil, from *Canning, Preserving and Pickling*, 1914

Marion Harris Neil was the "cookery editor" for the Ladies Home Journal *at the beginning of the twentieth century and wrote an entire book on chutneys, ketchups, and relishes! Elderberry chutney is one of those items that turns up again and again in historical cookbooks with extremely vague directions and ingredient lists. This is one of the easier to follow.* **Makes a couple small jars per pound of berries**

Elderberries
Onions
Cloves
Ground ginger
Brown sugar
Stoned raisins (i.e., seedless)
Red pepper
Mace
Salt
Mustard Seeds
Vinegar

For every pound of elderberries, allow 1 small onion, 8 cloves, ¼ ounce of ground ginger, ¼ pound of stoned raisins, a dust of red pepper and mace, ½ teaspoonful of mustard seeds, 1 teaspoonful of salt, and 1 cupful of vinegar.

Pound the berries and other ingredients together, then place them in an enameled pan, and boil for 10 minutes.

Remove from the fire, cover down, and leave until cold.

Divide into wide-mouthed bottles and cork down tightly.

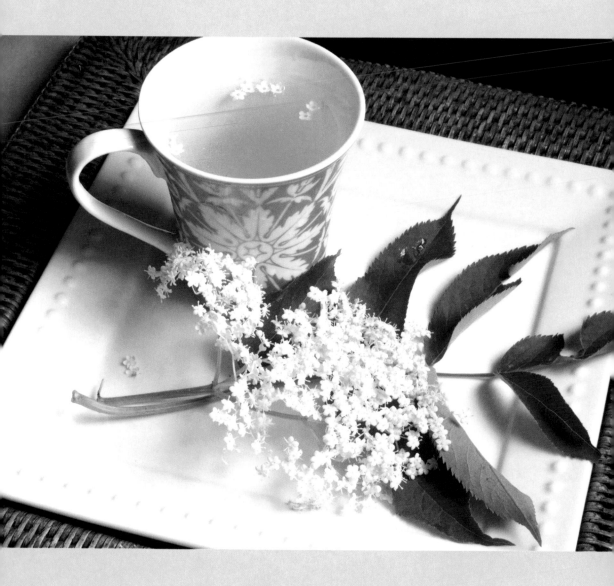

PART III:
ELDERBERRY AND
ELDERFLOWER DRINKS

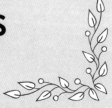

Easy Elderberry Spritzer

A healthy alternative to soda, elderberry spritzer is a refreshing, cooling drink that's a snap to make. You can use store-bought seltzer, but I strongly recommend making your own with a home carbonator, which saves quite a bit of money and plastic if you drink a lot of sparkling water. Because you can use filtered water and it's not steeping in a plastic bottle or plastic-lined can, you'll also have a far less chemical-laden beverage. **Makes 1 cup**

1 cup sparkling water or seltzer
2 tablespoons Elderberry Base (page 101)
Stevia or other sweetener to taste

Combine elderberry base and sparkling water, plus sweetener if desired. Serve over ice with a slice of lime.

You can also use elderberry syrup, but it makes a *very* sweet soda.

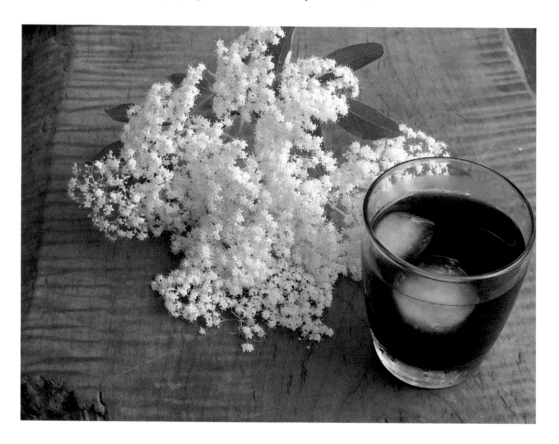

Sparkling Elderflower Soda

This light and simple soda made of seltzer and elderflower syrup is fantastic on its own or as a base for your favorite cocktail. Syrups you buy or make will vary quite a bit in sweetness and intensity of flavor, so use these amounts as starting points and adjust according to taste. **Makes 1 quart**

1 quart sparkling water or seltzer
¼ cup Elderflower Syrup (page 123)

Combine ingredients and taste.

Add more syrup if needed.

Serve over ice with a slice of lemon.

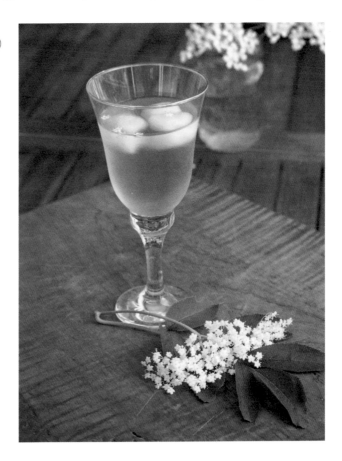

Fermented Elderberry and Honey Soda

Ariana Mullins, And Here We Are

This elderberry and honey soda is great to have around during cold and flu season, as both the honey and the elderberries have anti-viral properties. This fermented soda is probiotic, so it's a very well-rounded, healthy drink for the whole family! **Makes 8 servings**

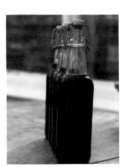

4 cups fresh elderberries (or 2 cups dried elderberries)
4 cups water
¾ cup raw, local honey or sugar (brown or sucanat would be nice)
Starter culture (like sauerkraut juice or whey from strained yogurt—
   you need 1–2 tablespoons)

Equipment needed: A demijohn, an airlock, a funnel, and swing-top bottles.

Put the elderberries into a pot, and add water. Bring to a simmer. Simmer for about 30 minutes over low heat, then cool.

Strain out the elderberries. Press with a spoon to extract as much juice as possible.

Add the sweetener to the remaining liquid and stir until dissolved. I used about ¾ cup, which made it very sweet. Keep in mind that the sugars will be digested by bacteria to create the fizz, so you do want to start with it much sweeter than you would like the soda to be.

Dilute the syrup with water to get a good juice flavor and consistency. Pour the "juice" into a sterilized or very clean demijohn, pour in your whey or sauerkraut juice, and add your airlock.

Let it sit for about 3 days, then taste it. Mine fermented pretty quickly, but there are some variables—the temperature of the room, the strength of the culture you used, etc. Taste it and let it ferment until it's only a little sweeter than you would like it to be.

Pour it into your swing-top bottles, and store in the fridge. (The type of bottle is important, as it allows the ferment to give off some small amounts of CO_2 and won't explode.) You could leave the soda out at room temperature if you'd like to drink it sooner, but I usually pop them into the fridge to slow down the fermentation process.

> **Notes:**
> - You will want to drink your soda within a few weeks, or you risk losing most of it to the "geyser effect." Check in now and then to see what kind of pressure is building up. Your beverage will get drier, more tart, and fizzier the longer you wait. It will eventually develop more of an alcohol content, too, so you might want to taste it before giving it to kids if you've been storing it for a while! Enjoy!

Elderberry-Infused Brandy, Gin, or Vodka (Elderberry Liqueur)

Liqueur is one of the simplest spirits to make, involving nothing more than steeping your berries or flowers in alcohol, like a tincture, but with sweetener added. This rich liqueur can be sipped medicinally, or enjoyed as an aperitif or cocktail mix-in. It also makes a great homemade gift! **Makes 2 to 3 cups**

2 cups fresh or frozen elderberries
3-inch strip of lemon peel, without pith
2–3 cups brandy, gin, or vodka
¼–½ cup sugar per quart alcohol, depending on how sweet you want the finished liqueur

Place berries and lemon peel in a quart jar and cover completely with alcohol.

Allow to sit and infuse 1–3 months in a cool, dark place. Longer steep times will result in a richer flavor. Strain out berries and lemon peel. Add sugar and stir. Allow to rest another week or so until sugar is fully dissolved.

Keeps indefinitely.

Note: Use a vegetable peeler to peel a whole lemon, making sure not to get any bitter pith. Alternatively, you can cut pieces of lemon peel and remove pith with a knife.

Borage Elderflower Tea

Borage is an underappreciated herb that's easy to grow and utterly delicious. Somehow its odd, fuzzy leaves are brimming with the flavor of melon and cucumber, and combined with elderflowers make a delicate and refreshing iced tea, celebrating the fresh tastes of summer. I like to make mine as a sun tea and enjoy with plenty of ice. **Makes 1 quart**

1 cup borage leaves and flowers
1 head elderflower blossoms,
    removed from stem
1 quart filtered water

Place borage and elderflowers in a 1-quart mason jar and cover with water. Screw on the lid and leave in the sun for at least 5 hours, longer if possible. Strain and serve over ice. For an extra-special twist, float borage flowers and elderflowers on top or freeze into ice cubes before serving.

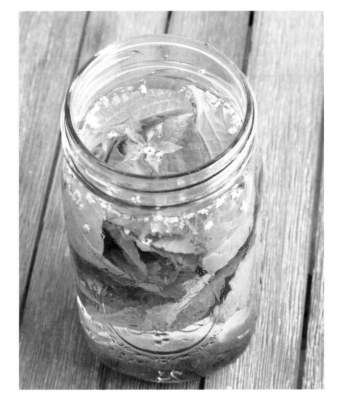

Elderflower Lemon Balm Iced Tea

Floral elderflower and bright lemon balm combine in this winning drink. I love to harness the power of the sun in summer and make sun teas when the herbs are plentiful in the garden. The flavor is less intense than when it's brewed with boiling water, but you also get to save energy and skip the heat of boiling water. Best served over ice in summer, you can also brew it with dried elderflower and lemon balm for a warming winter brew that's good for fighting off viruses and promoting sleep. **Makes 1 quart**

2 generous cups loose-packed fresh lemon balm (or 2 tablespoons dried)
1 large elderflower head (or 2 tablespoons dried)
3 cups filtered water

If using fresh herbs, harvest in the morning.

Rinse the lemon balm and place in a clean quart mason jar or large tea pot.

Pull the blossoms from the elderflower head and add to the jar.

Add boiled filtered water and stir to combine.

Infuse at least 10 minutes, but preferably several hours.

If making sun tea:

- Use a mason jar and fill with cold water. Screw on lid, and turn upside down to mix. Place in sun for at least 8 hours.
- Strain and serve over ice with a garnish of fresh lemon balm or a slice of lemon. Sweeten if desired.

Hibiscus Elderflower Tea

Hibiscus elderflower tea is a delicious, antioxidant-rich drink. Hibiscus has an impressive array of health benefits of its own, including lowering blood pressure and cholesterol and improving metabolism. Hibiscus brews up a gorgeous red and makes a refreshingly tart tea. Elderflower adds extra floral notes. This combo makes a healthy replacement for juice drinks and other sweetened beverages, though it's recommended to consume hibiscus in moderation because of its powerful effects on the body. (See cautions below.) **Makes 2 cups**

2 cups boiled filtered water
1 tablespoon loose hibiscus
1½ teaspoons dried elderflower
1 drop liquid stevia or other sweetener to taste (optional)

Add boiled water to hibiscus and elderflower in a teapot or infuser cup.

Steep at least 10 minutes and up to several hours, or brew as a sun tea. Strain and add sweetener if desired. Best served over lots of ice.

A few cautions with hibiscus:

- Pregnant women should avoid hibiscus as it may induce premature labor.
- Because hibiscus is often intercropped with peanuts, people with severe peanut allergies may react to hibiscus.
- Avoid hibiscus if you are on blood pressure–lowering medication and talk to your doctor before consuming hibiscus if you are on other medications or have health issues.

Rhubarb Elderberry Cooler

This refreshing summer drink is the perfect way to make use of the gorgeous pink liquid left over when you strain the rhubarb cooked for making Elderberry Rhubarb Fruit Leather (page 138). For years I threw it away, until I discovered it made a fantastic add-in to things like lemonade, or even on its own with a little sweetener. This cooler combines the bright, tart flavor of rhubarb with the darker flavor of elderberry and is just perfect on a hot summer day served over ice. **Makes 1 to 2 servings**

1 cup rhubarb "juice" (see details below)
3 tablespoons Elderberry Base (page 101) or Simple Elderberry Syrup (page 102)
Still or sparkling water
Sweetener to taste (I use a squirt of liquid stevia per glass)

This recipe is a little inexact, in large part because the rhubarb juice will vary in intensity depending on how much water the rhubarb cooked in when you made your fruit leather. If you're not making leather, you can also brew up a simple rhubarb juice by simmering a pound of rhubarb in 4 cups water and straining the solids out. (But I highly recommend using that rhubarb for leather—it's unbelievably good!)

Add elderberry concentrate to rhubarb juice and dilute with water to taste. Sweeten if desired. Serve over ice.

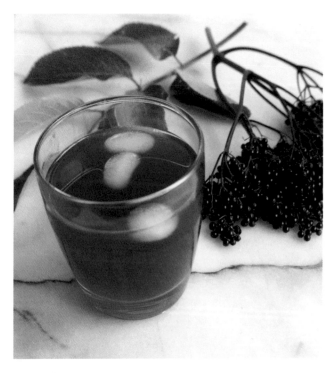

Elderflower Champagne Fizz

Carol Little, Studio Botanica

Elderflower "fizz" is a delightful remedy/libation/afternoon sipping beverage from "way back." I first tasted it in Provence, France, in 2003 during a "Plant Lover's Journey" with my dear friend and mentor, Rosemary Gladstar. What a delightful trip; so full of the wonder of the plants! The glorious afternoon was only made more perfect by the arrival of elderflower champagne and subsequent sipping! This, of course, is not really a champagne, nor is it alcoholic, but it is a refreshing and deliciously fragrant drink to serve on a summer's day. **Makes about 1 gallon**

1 gallon filtered water
¾ cup sugar (organic cane sugar, coconut sugar, or favorite sweetener)
2 organic lemons
4 large elderflower heads (or more)
2 tablespoons white wine vinegar or rice vinegar

Boil the water, then stir in the sugar until it has dissolved, and leave to cool.

Zest both lemons.

Extract juice from one lemon and cut the other lemon into slices.

Place the elderflowers in a large, non-metallic container.

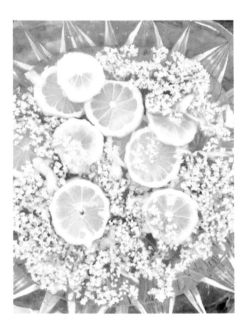

Add the lemon zest, juice, and slices, the sweetened water, and the vinegar.

Stir, cover with a cloth, and leave for 24 hours.

Strain the liquid through a fine sieve, squeezing the flowers to extract all the flavor.

Pour into clean screw-top or swing-top bottles.

Store, preferably on their sides, for 10 days, until effervescent.

Drink within 3 to 4 weeks.

Elderberry Switchel

Haven't quite gotten around to brewing your own kombucha? Making a hip fermented drink is as simple as mixing a few simple ingredients for a tangy and delicious homemade drink called a switchel. A go-to refresher in the days before soda and energy drinks, the acidity of the vinegar and the spicy ginger flavor pair well with elderberry syrup. You can try spiced or plain syrup, or use unsweetened elderberry base if you prefer. Traditionally served over ice to cool off on hot days, it's also delicious at room temperature even when it's not hot out. This combo of ginger, honey, probiotics, and elderberry is also great for immune support. **Makes 3 servings**

3 cups filtered water
2 tablespoons organic unfiltered apple cider vinegar
2 tablespoons raw honey
1 tablespoon fresh ginger root, peeled and chopped
½ cup Simple Elderberry Syrup (page 102)

Combine all ingredients in a jar or pitcher, and allow to steep at room temperature for at least a few hours.

Strain and serve plain or over ice.

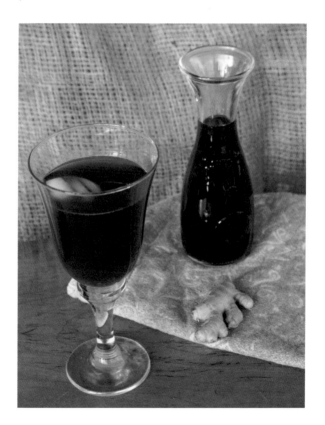

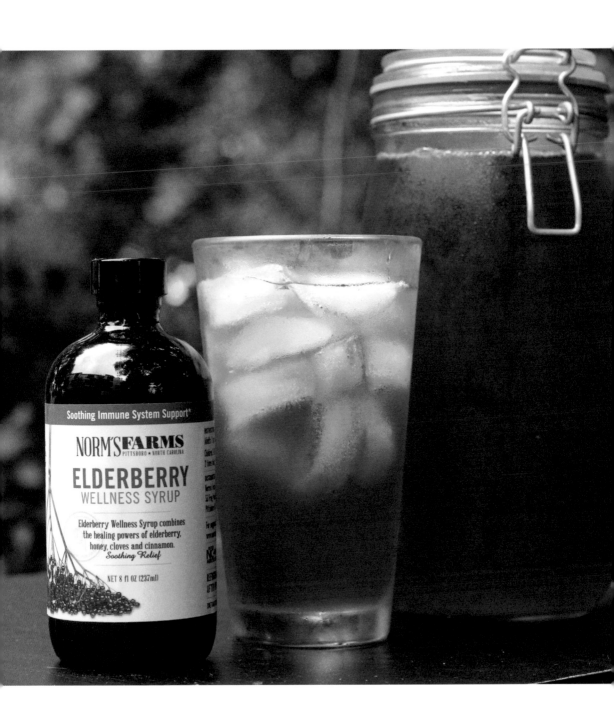

Elderberry Kombucha

Ann Lenhardt, Norm's Farms

The Chinese referred to kombucha as an "Immortal Health Elixir." Kombucha is a fermented beverage made with black tea, sugar, and water. The fermentation is caused by a colony of bacteria and yeast commonly known as a SCOBY, which stands for "symbiotic colony of bacteria and yeast." Kombucha is refreshing and delicious, and best of all, it is also a functional, probiotic food with great health benefits. This recipe includes elderberry syrup for an extra immune system boost and incredible flavor. **Makes 3½ quarts**

1 gallon spring water
1 cup pure cane sugar
1 ounce loose black or green tea, or 3 tea bags
SCOBY with Starter Tea
Norm's Farms Elderberry Syrup (or see page 102)

Equipment:
1-gallon size fermenting jar
2 (2-quart) glass second fermentation jars with flip-top lids
Clean kitchen towel or cheese cloth and a rubber band

Sterilize the 1-gallon size fermenting jar with hot soapy water, rinse well in hot water, and allow to dry.

Bring ½ gallon spring water to boil. Combine hot water and sugar in a large glass bowl and stir until sugar is dissolved.

Add tea and allow to steep 35 to 40 minutes. Remove tea bags, if using, or strain loose tea from liquid by pouring the liquid through a fine mesh sieve.

Pour concentrated sweet tea mixture into sterilized gallon fermentation vessel.

Top off with ½ gallon cool spring water.

Check the temperature of the tea. When it has completely cooled to room temperature, add the SCOBY and a bit of starter tea that it came with.

Place a clean dishcloth or cheese cloth over the opening of the fermentation vessel and secure with a rubber band.

Allow to sit for 7 to 10 days. On day 7, test the kombucha with a straw. If the kombucha is too sweet for your liking, allow it to sit for a day or two more and then test again. You want to find a balance between not too sweet and not too sour.

(continued on next page)

Clean and sanitize the 2-quart jars with flip-top lids, being sure to clean the gaskets that create the air-tight seal. Allow to air dry.

Pour 7 to 7½ cups of kombucha liquid through a fine mesh sieve into each of the 2-quart jars, reserving 1 to 2 cups of tea and the "mother" SCOBY in the gallon fermentation vessel.

Add 1 to 2 ounces of elderberry syrup to the kombucha in each of the 2-quart jars. The amount you add depends on your flavor preference, so go ahead and taste it after adding one ounce. If you want a stronger flavor, add another ounce.

Tightly close each jar and let ferment another 2 to 4 days.

Important: As the kombucha feeds on the added sugar, CO_2 will build up in the jars so it is important that you "burp" the jars once a day by briefly opening them.

This is the time to get your next batch of kombucha brewing! Repeat steps 1 through 8 with the reserved SCOBY and starter tea.

On day 2 taste the kombucha in the second fermentation vessels to determine if it's fizzy enough and tastes the way you like it. The longer you let it ferment, the less sweet it will become. If you find the kombucha too sweet, allow it to ferment another day, and taste again.

When the kombucha has achieved the flavor you want, place both glass jars in the refrigerator to stop the fermentation process.

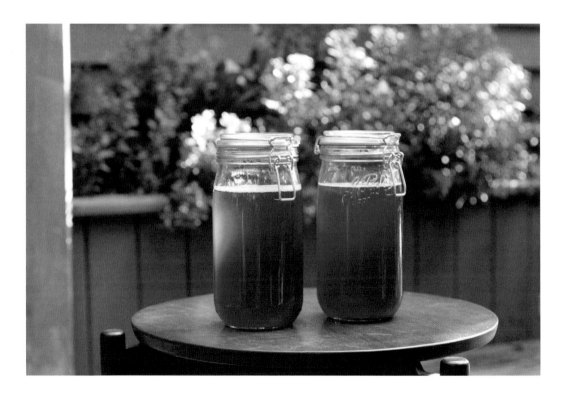

Notes:

- It's fine if your mother SCOBY sinks to the bottom. A SCOBY baby will form at the surface too. As your SCOBY reproduces, pass the babies along to your friends with some starter tea so that they can make their own kombucha too. Brown spots, stringy stuff, and floaties are all normal. These can be strained before drinking, but don't worry if you consume some of it—it's just yeast and it's good for you!

- However, mold can form on the surface of your kombucha and that is *not* good for you. You'll know it is mold because it is fuzzy and blue-green, green, or grey, just like mold that grows on bread or cheese, and it really doesn't look like the SCOBY. If mold has formed on the surface of your kombucha, your SCOBY is ruined and must be discarded. To prevent mold, maintain proper ratios of tea, water, and sugar. Herbal teas are not recommended because they don't always contain the food the SCOBY requires. Stick with black and green teas when getting started. You can use Oolong or White tea when your SCOBY is well established (you've made several batches of kombucha). Keep your fermenting kombucha out of direct sunlight and in a steady temperature environment for best results.

Elderflower Liqueur

Known as "bartender's salt" or "bartender's ketchup" because of its go-to flavor for cocktails, this sweet liqueur is a staple in numerous drinks (some included below), and according to Loon Liquor's Simeon Rossi, makes just about any drink memorable. "It tastes like a summer breeze going down a country road," he told me as we de-stemmed flowers that he would transform into the popular liqueur. He says that when customers try it in Loon Liquor's cocktail room, they often purchase a bottle to take home. They're fascinated it by it, he says, because elderflower "is not part of their mental flavor bank." Add it to yours! **Makes 1 quart**

10–20 elderflower heads
1 quart 80- or 100-proof vodka
¼ cup organic cane sugar

De-stem your flowers carefully, removing as much of the green stem as possible. Fill a clean glass jar with the de-stemmed flowers and cover completely with vodka. You can use fermentation weights to hold down the flowers, which may oxidize and turn brown if they float to the top.

Cap the jar and allow to sit for 1 week for a milder flavor and up to 1 month for a stronger one.

Strain out the flowers using a fine sieve lined with cloth.

Add sugar, shaking to dissolve. You can add more sugar if you prefer a sweeter liqueur.

Notes:

- Fresh flowers are best for this project. When Rossi made a test batch with dried flowers he found the result "papery" and thoroughly unpalatable, though I have seen recipes that call for either fresh or dried flowers.
- Rossi recommends 67 grams of flower blossoms per quart of vodka, but you can also use the folk method and nearly fill a jar with blossoms, then cover with vodka.

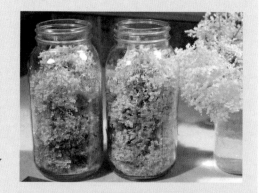

Elderflower Sangria

Traditionally, sangria is made with red wine and citrus fruit, but there's no reason your sangria has to be traditional! Have some fun mixing things up with different seasonal fruits, wines, and other add-ins. Use peaches and berries, pineapple or pomegranate, and use plenty of elderflower liqueur to give it that special sparkle. It all comes together in the pitcher, getting better as it sits. **Makes approx. 1 quart**

1 orange, sliced or cut in wedges
1 lemon, sliced or cut in wedges
1 lime, sliced or cut in wedges
¾ cup orange juice (plus more to taste)
⅓ cup Elderflower Liqueur (page 164)
750-ml bottle dry red wine (white wine
    works also)

Optional:
2 cups seltzer water
¼ cup brandy

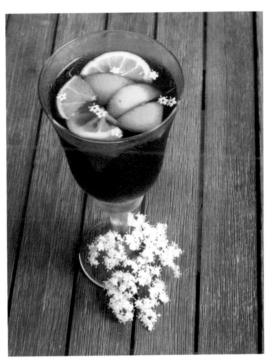

Add all ingredients to a pitcher and stir to combine.

Allow to chill in the refrigerator at least 1 hour, more if possible.

Serve straight or over ice. Garnish with fruit if desired.

Store in the refrigerator. Flavors will continue to meld with time. Best consumed in a few days.

If you like your sangria sweeter, a little elderflower syrup would add sweetness as well as more elderflower flavor.

Sun-Extracted Elderberry Wine

Laurie Neverman, Commonsense Home

You, too, can be "feeling fine on elderberry wine," as the Elton John song goes. This easy elderberry wine has just four ingredients and brews in the sun. The recipe is adapted from the 1979 book How to Make Wine in Your Own Kitchen *by Mettja Cappon Roate.* **Makes about 3 (750-ml) bottles**

4 quarts loosely packed dark, ripe elderberries
2 quarts water
6 cups cane sugar
1 cup chopped raisins

This recipe is made in stages. In stage one, you steep the elderberries in water; in stage two, you add the sugar and raisins.

Pack your elderberries into a gallon glass jar. Bring 2 quarts of water to a boil. Make sure your jar is warm (you can set it in a tub of warm water) to prevent breakage. Pour the boiling water over the elderberries. Leave an inch of space at the top, because they will swell and expand.

Make a plastic liner for the metal cover. Put the cover on loosely (tight enough to keep bugs out, but loose enough that it can vent). Set in a sunny place outside for 3 days, after which the liquid should be bright red in color. Strain the berries through a jelly bag or flour sack towel, squeezing out as much liquid as possible.

Pour juice back into the glass jar or 1-gallon crock. Stir in the sugar, making sure it is all dissolved. Add chopped raisins.

Cover loosely and keep in a warm place indoors to continue fermentation for 3 more weeks.

At the end of this time period, strain through several layers of cheesecloth (a flour sack towel or old, clean cotton T-shirt will also work). Siphon into clean, sterilized bottles.

Cork lightly at first (or put a balloon over the top). When your balloon doesn't inflate or you see no bubbles on the bottle walls, cork tightly and store on their sides. Seal with wax for longer storage. Keep for at least 1 year before drinking.

Notes:
- You'll notice this recipe has no added yeast. This made me a little nervous, since wild yeast can be less reliable. If you don't see bubbles within a couple days, it's probably safer to add commercial yeast so your wine doesn't spoil or turn into vinegar.

Chokecherry Elderflower Mead

Chris Dalziel, Joybilee Farm

Honey mead is fermented wine sweetened with honey instead of sugar. It contains all the healthy elements of the honey as well as healthful probiotics. Honey mead traditionally was used as medicine, preserving the medicinal benefits of herbs into the winter.

Chokecherries are rich in antioxidants. Elderflowers, too, help fight winter colds and flu symptoms. This honey mead will preserve the goodness of summer herbs and fruit for winter. Honey mead making is very forgiving. You don't need to measure exactly. If you don't have access to chokecherries, black or wild cherries may be used. Dried elderflowers can also take the place of fresh. **Makes 5 (750 ml) bottles**

1 cup fresh elderflowers, de-stemmed (or ½ cup dried)
½ cup fresh rose petals
8–10 cups filtered water, divided
3 cups honey
6 pounds chokecherries, or 6 cups chokecherry juice
½ cup grape juice concentrate
¼ teaspoon champagne wine yeast

Equipment:
One glass gallon jug and one fermentation lock for each batch of mead you want to make, plus one extra glass gallon jug for siphoning off the mead when you are ready to rack it
Food-safe siphon hose
5 wine bottles with corks or caps to hold your finished wine
Wine bottle corker

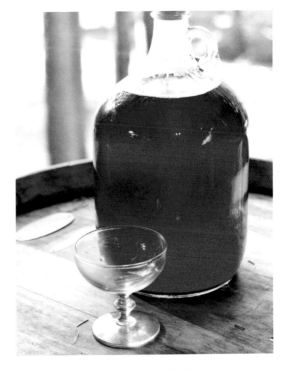

Place elderflowers and rose petals in a 2-quart, heat-proof bowl. Pour 4 cups boiling water over them and let steep for 1 hour, covered. Strain, and stir in the honey. Set aside.

Meanwhile, remove the stems from the chokecherries and place them in a steam juicer. Steam until the juice flows freely. If you don't have a steam juicer, simmer the cherries in a pot with 2 cups of water for 30 minutes until cherries are steaming.

(continued on next page)

Strain through a jelly bag or through cheesecloth, squeezing to extract as much juice as possible. The juice will be cloudy but will clear during the fermentation process. Reserve the juice. Discard the pulp and seeds.

Sanitize a 1-gallon glass fermenting jug, along with its tin cap. Pour the herb and honey mixture into the fermenting jug. Add the chokecherry juice.

Pour the grape juice concentrate into a glass. Stir in 1 cup water, and allow to come to room temperature. Sprinkle the yeast over top of the grape juice. Wait 30 minutes. Stir the yeast into the grape juice and wait till it becomes frothy or bubbly.

Pour the grape juice-yeast mixture into the fermentation jug. Cap the jug and shake it for a few minutes to finish dissolving both the yeast and the honey. Add the cooled honey-herb tea to the fermentation jug. Top up the jug to the shoulders with boiled and cooled filtered water.

Sanitize a wine fermentation lock. Fill the fermentation lock with boiled and cooled water. Replace the cap on the fermentation jug with the fermentation lock.

Place the jug on a plate to catch any overflow and put in a spot out of direct sunlight and away from sources of heat for several weeks. The fermentation will become active with bubbling and frothing evident.

Racking off:

After 4 to 6 weeks you'll notice that the fermentation has slowed down and sediment is forming in the bottom of the jug. The mead won't be clear though. When the bubbling and frothing stop, transfer the liquid to a fresh, sanitized fermentation jug. Sanitize the fermentation lock again and place it on the new fermentation jug. The fermentation process will resume.

Clear the mead:

This last fermentation can take anywhere from 2 to 6 weeks. When the fermentation stops, the wine will clear. If it doesn't clear naturally, add ¼ teaspoon of pectinase to the jug. Replace the fermentation lock and wait.

Bottle the mead:

When the wine clears and fermentation stops, siphon the mead into sanitized wine bottles. Cap with a wine corker or a twist cap according to your bottles. Label the bottles.

Place the wine bottles in a cool, dark spot. Age at least 3 months before sampling. Mead gets better the longer it sits.

Midcilantro Night's Dream

Simeon Rossi, Loon Liquor

One of Loon Liquor's most popular cocktails, this unusual drink is full of surprises, especially the little kick of hot pepper at the end. **Makes 1 cocktail**

2 ounces Wheaton Barley Vodka
1 ounce spicy ginger soda
½ ounce Elderflower Lac Coeur (or homemade Elderflower Liqueur, see page 164)
½ ounce fresh lime juice
½ ounce lime simple syrup (instructions below)
4–6 drops serrano pepper tincture (instructions below)
1 bunch (roughly 12) cilantro leaves

Add all ingredients to an ice-filled shaker and shake until chilled.

Double strain into a chilled lowball glass.

Garnish with a cilantro sprig and lime twist.

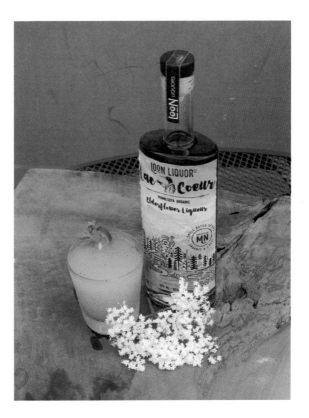

Notes:
- To make a lime simple syrup: Combine 1 cup cane sugar and 1 cup water, and bring to a boil, stirring until all sugar is dissolved. Remove sugar solution from heat, add the zest of 5 limes, and let rest for 15 minutes. Strain and refrigerate.
- Serrano pepper tincture: Combine ½ cup vodka and 2 tablespoons red pepper flakes in a clean jar and allow to rest 1 month. Strain and transfer to a dropper bottle.

Elderflower Punch with Turmeric
(Punch Fleur de Sureau/Curcuma)

Bertrand Bouflet, La Maison du Sureau

La Maison du Sureau celebrates the joys of experimenting with all things elderberry (and elderflower), and this cocktail combines their goodness in one drink. An amazing (and medicinal) cocktail like no other! **Makes 4 to 5 servings**

8½ ounces water
2 teaspoons turmeric powder
2 tablespoons dried elderflower
3 tablespoons Simple Elderberry Syrup (page 102)
1 fresh apple
Juice of half a lemon
4 mint leaves, minced
3 tablespoons + 1 teaspoon Elderflower Liqueur (page 164)
Sparkling water

Bring the water to a boil. Place the turmeric and the dried elderflower in a teapot or infuser cup, and add boiling water. Infuse for 5 minutes.

Strain, then add the elderberry syrup and chill.

Peel and seed the apple and cut it into thin slices.

Take chilled turmeric elderflower infusion and add lemon juice, apple, minced mint leaves, and elderflower liqueur. Mix well.

Pour in glasses with a little sparkling water and ice.

Hugo Cocktail

Bertrand Bouflet, La Maison du Sureau

This popular cocktail is simple, but so delicious that it's in high demand in much of Europe during the summer. Originally made with lemon balm syrup, elderflower syrup or liqueur has become a staple ingredient in this well-loved drink. **Makes 1 cocktail**

2 tablespoons Elderflower Liqueur (page 164)
3⅓ ounces sparkling water
5 ounces sparkling wine (such as Prosecco, Champagne, or Crément)
3–4 fresh mint leaves
1 slice of lime
4–5 ice cubes

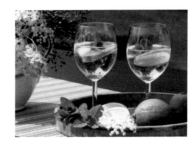

Pour liqueur, sparkling water, and Prosecco into a large wine glass.

Add the fresh mint leaves and lime.

Add ice cubes and stir gently with a spoon for 8 to 10 seconds to combine before serving.

Notes:

- You can also make a "Virgin Hugo" without alcohol by replacing the Prosecco with lemonade or sparkling water and using 60 ml of elderflower syrup in place of the liqueur.

PART IV:
ELDER FOR SKIN CARE (AND OTHER THINGS, TOO)

If you're into DIY beauty, you'll love working elderflowers into your homemade skin care products. Prized for their skin-soothing and skin-smoothing abilities, elderflowers make wonderful additions to moisturizers and salves.

Elderflower Rose Hip Salve

Jan Berry, The Nerdy Farm Wife

This salve features elderflowers, an old-fashioned remedy for softer, more evenly toned skin. Elderflowers are also traditionally used to heal scrapes, scratches, and wounds, and as a treatment for dry skin. I like to include rose hip seed oil in this salve, for its well-known effectiveness against scarring, wrinkles, and signs of aging. **Makes 4 ounces**

¼ cup dried elderflower
½ cup sunflower, sweet almond, or other oil
½ ounce (14 grams) beeswax
½ ounce (14 grams) rose hip seed oil
1 vitamin E capsule (optional)

If you don't have rose hip seed oil, you may use more elderflower-infused oil in its place.

First, place dried elderflowers in a small jar and add oil.

For a quick infusion: Set the uncovered jar down into a small saucepan filled with a few inches of water. Heat over a low burner for 1 to 2 hours, making sure that the water doesn't evaporate out. Remove from heat and strain.

For a slower, more traditional infusion: Cap the jar and tuck away in a cabinet for around 4 to 6 weeks, shaking occasionally. When the infusing time has passed, strain.

You can also set the jar in a sunny windowsill for several days to a week to jump-start the infusion. Don't store for long periods in sunlight though, as it tends to fade flowers and herbs over time.

Measure your strained oil. You'll need 3 ounces (85 grams) of elderflower-infused oil. Any leftover can be used as a simple moisturizing oil. You may also re-use the elderflowers to infuse more oil for additional projects.

Combine the elderflower-infused oil and beeswax in a heat-proof container, like a canning jar or Pyrex pitcher. Set the container down into a pan filled with a few inches of water, forming a makeshift double boiler.

Place the pan over low heat until the beeswax melts. Remove from heat and stir in the rose hip seed oil. You can squeeze the contents of a vitamin E capsule into the salve to help lengthen shelf life. You can also add a few drops of essential oil, such as lavender or rose, if you'd like your salve to be scented.

Pour into tins or jars and allow to cool completely.

To use: Apply a thin light layer to hands, face, and throat at night. This salve is best suited for those with dry and/or mature skin.

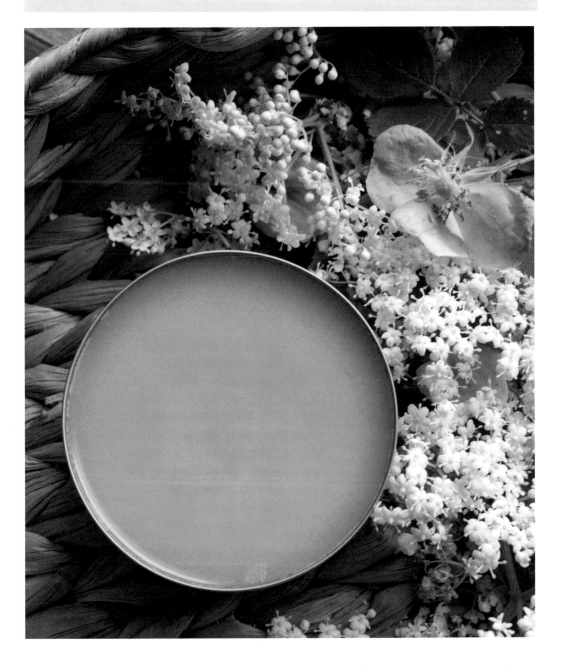

Anti-Aging Elderflower Salve

Vladka Merva, Simply Beyond Herbs

Both elderflower and frankincense oil have positive effects on older skin and prevent signs of aging, making this salve ideal for mature skin. **Makes approx. 4 ounces**

½ cup elderflower-infused oil (page 178)
2 tablespoons beeswax (or candelilla wax for vegan option)
15 drops frankincense essential oil

Place the elderflower-infused oil and beeswax in a double boiler. Gently heat the mixture just until the beeswax has melted.

As soon as the wax is melted, remove from heat.

Allow it to cool slightly, and stir in frankincense essential oil.

Fill your salve container when the mixture is still liquid.

Let it set for 2 hours before using.

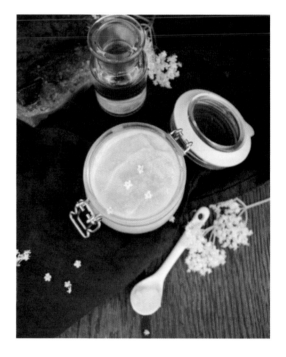

Notes:
- Salves can last for 1 to 3 years if stored properly. They should be stored in a cool place or refrigerator. Make sure they don't re-melt and re-solidify as this will hinder their medicinal properties.
- You can use fresh elderflowers in the oil if you prefer, but infused oils from dried herbs tend to last longer.

Elderflower Lip Balm

Vladka Merva, Simply Beyond Herbs

There are several advantages to making your own lip balm. You'll likely save money, and you can reuse plastic tubes, making your lip balm more sustainable. You also get to control the ingredients and can avoid chemical-filled products. This easy softening lip balm with elderflower is a great place to start. **Makes 4 tubes**

2 tablespoons elderflower-infused oil (page 178)
1 tablespoon beeswax
1 tablespoon coconut oil

Gently heat the elderflower-infused oil in a double boiler with the beeswax and coconut oil.

Stir until the beeswax and coconut oil are fully melted.

Fill the lip balm tubes or a small jar when still warm.

Note: You can adjust the hardness and viscosity of the balm by playing with the quantity ratio of beeswax and coconut oil. If you prefer softer, you can add more coconut oil, and if you prefer harder, more beeswax.

Elder Leaf Salve

Jan Berry, The Nerdy Farm Wife

The idea for this elder leaf salve came from one of my all-time favorite books, Making Plant Medicine, *by Richo Cech. He states that oils and salves made from fresh elder leaves "make a useful application to traumatic injuries, old burns, ulcerations, or hemorrhoids." Kiva Rose, another highly respected herbalist, says: "Infused oil of the flowers or leaves makes a wonderful salve or ointment for all kinds of wounds, as well as bruises, sprains, and strains."* **Makes 3 (2-ounce) tins**

¼ cup elder leaves
⅔ cup sunflower, sweet almond, or other oil
½ ounce (14 grams) beeswax

You'll first need to infuse your oil.

Normally, I shy away from making infused oils with freshly picked leaves or flowers, because the added water content tends to make them spoil more easily. Since elder leaves are abundant and free for the picking, though, I've tried it both ways. I found that the fresh leaf method made a much greener (and theoretically more potent) salve, but I still prefer using wilted leaves, for a less-cloudy and longer-lasting oil infusion. Feel free to use whichever method you prefer.

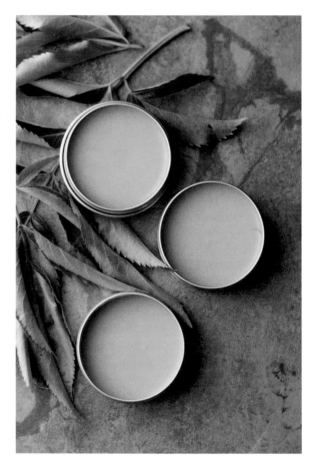

Wilted leaf method: Gather a handful of elder leaves and spread them out in a single layer overnight or up to 24 hours, until wilted and almost dry. Place the leaves in a glass canning jar and cover with oil.

Fresh leaf method: Gather a handful of leaves and place them in a jar. Cover the leaves with oil.

Set the uncovered jar into a saucepan filled with a few inches of water, forming a makeshift double-boiler. Place the pan over a low burner and heat the oil for around 2 hours. Keep a close eye on things to make sure that the water doesn't evaporate out of the pan.

After the infusing time is up, you can strain the oil and proceed with the recipe right away or you can cover the jar with a piece of cheesecloth or scrap of old, clean t-shirt (so any remaining moisture has room to escape) and let the oil infuse for several days, or even weeks. If using fresh leaves, it's best to let the strained oil settle out overnight and then carefully pour the good oil out, leaving behind the sludgy layer that settles to the bottom.

Place 3½ ounces (100 grams) of the oil and the beeswax in a canning jar or heat-proof container. Set the jar down into a saucepan containing a few inches of water, forming a makeshift double boiler.

Set the pan over medium-low heat until the beeswax is melted. If you used a small canning jar for melting, you can use it for storing the salve as well.

Notes:
- Elder leaf–infused oil would also work in a balm for aches and pains, but since the leaves have compounds which are toxic when ingested, avoid using it in lip balms, nursing balms, or on young children or people who may inadvertently rub some in their mouth. In short, don't eat the leaves!
- I recommend using a digital scale to make all of your herbal and cosmetic products, but I know not everyone has one handy. If you'd like to make this by volume, the beeswax converts to roughly 1½ tablespoons (grated or pastilles, packed very tightly in the spoon) and the oil measures out to be approximately ½ cup. You might need to tinker with the amounts of oil and beeswax, remelting the salve as needed, to get a consistency that you like.

Elderberry Ink, Watercolor, and Dye

I was intrigued by the uses of elderberry as an ink and dye, so my daughter and I read up on berry-based inks and experimented with some elderberries we had left over from other projects. Elderberry ink comes out a lovely reddish-purple color. Note that it will fade readily if exposed to sunlight and does not keep long. **Makes approx. ¼ cup**

1 large head very ripe elderberries
Salt
White vinegar

Remember, elderberry's juice makes a good dye and ink because it *stains*! Dress appropriately, and use only metal, ceramic, and glass equipment.

Options for preparing the berries:

Simmering the berries briefly and mashing them will help to extract the juice and concentrate it, producing a darker ink that may keep better, but you can skip this step if you want to make a lighter ink that's probably better to use as a watercolor. If you want to make a dark ink, I recommend cooking.

Popping your berries in the freezer for a while will make destemming and extracting juice from your berries easier, but it's not absolutely necessary. Some sources suggest macerating mashed berries in a little water with a black tea bag for a day or so instead.

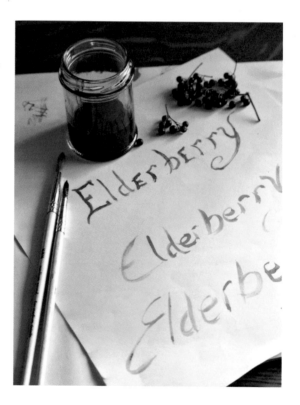

To extract the juice: Put a sieve over a large bowl and put de-stemmed berries in. We used scissors to remove most of the stem and didn't bother carefully de-stemming all of them. If using frozen berries, allow them to thaw before mashing.

The easiest way to extract the juice is by pushing the berries through the sieve with a large spoon. You can line the sieve with cheesecloth or fabric, or strain the juice a second time using a cloth or jelly bag, or even some old tights. Some sources recommend using a mortar and pestle to crush the berries before pushing them through the strainer.

To make the ink: Measure the juice you've extracted. For every ¼ cup, add ¼ teaspoon of salt and ½ teaspoon of white vinegar. Stir to combine. Alternatively, you can use powdered gum arabic and alum, about 2 grams each for each cup of liquid.

If you'd like the color to concentrate further, leave it to evaporate a day or so. Use quickly, as it doesn't keep well. We stored ours in the refrigerator to prolong its usable life.

Remember that elderberry was also used to dye hair and clothing. If you try an elderberry paste on your hair, do let me know how it works!

To use elderberry as a clothing dye: Simmer berries in twice as much water for an hour, while simmering the cloth to be dyed in 4 cups of water with ¼ cup salt. Strain the berry water. Rinse the clothing well and allow to soak in the berry dye until you get the desired color. Wash in cold water. Elderberry leaves and bark can also be used to dye cloth green or grey.

Elder Leaf
Pest Repellent & Fertilizer

The compounds that make the leaves unsafe to eat make them useful for repelling garden pests. As I've mentioned, S. canadensis *leaves have very little of the smell* S. nigra *is famous for, so they may not work as well as nigra-based concoctions. I confirmed with Bertrand Bouflet of La Maison du Sureau, who uses a common recipe for fermented elder leaf extract in his own garden, that the smell is indeed very powerful and unpleasant, but also very effective.* **Makes approx. 1 liter**

Elder leaf decoction (*décoction de sureau*): Soak 100 grams of fresh elderberry leaves in 1 liter of rain water for 24 hours. Simmer 30 minutes, and allow to cool. Strain and pour into a spray bottle. Use undiluted on leaves and around the base of plants to deter insects and rodents. It's reported to be especially effective against aphids, flea beetles, moths, voles, and moles.

Fermented elder leaf extract (*purin de sureau*): Chop 100 grams of fresh elderberry leaves and soak in 1 liter of rain water for 6 to 8 days, stirring daily. Keep in a shaded place, ideally between 59 and 73°F. You will see bubbles from the fermentation process. When they stop, your extract is ready to strain.

Pour into a spray bottle, diluting to 10% with water if using as a fertilizer. Bouflet recommends diluting to 25% if using as a pest-repellent and antifungal.

I would advise not using this spray on leaves you plan to eat, like salad greens and spinach. While it might help with aphids and flea beetles, I would be concerned about being able to get all the extract off before eating. But as a spray on the leaves of fruiting plants there should be less to worry about as long as you avoid spraying the fruit itself.

You can also try simply spreading bruised or crumbled leaves around plants you want to protect.

Bouflet also says elder leaves can help accelerate the composting process.

CONTRIBUTORS

Ashley Adamant lives in rural Vermont with her husband and two small children. You can find her work at PracticalSelfReliance.com, where she shares detailed tutorials for gardening, foraging, and all things DIY, and at AdamantKitchen.com, where she shares her favorite recipes.

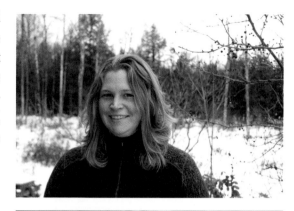

Belvoir Fruit Farms have been making the United Kingdom's finest cordials and ready-to-drink, lightly sparkling pressés for thirty-five years. Still a family-owned and run business, they remain true to their roots, with their whole range made on the farm using only the finest natural ingredients and no artificial sweeteners, flavorings, colorings, or preservatives. They are best known for their Elderflower Cordial, using a family recipe made mainly from elderflowers grown in the company's ninety acres of elderflower plantations (the only ones in the UK) and from bushes growing wild in the hedgerows. Locals help bring the harvest home each year in a race against time; the season lasts just six short weeks. Pev, son of the cordial's originator Mary Manners, says, "Every bottle of Belvoir Elderflower Cordial contains about eight elderflower heads, and each summer we make enough bottles to last the year. We need around 3.6 million flowerheads each harvest to keep up with demand; that's a lot of elderflowers and a lot of work but we hope you agree it's worth it!"

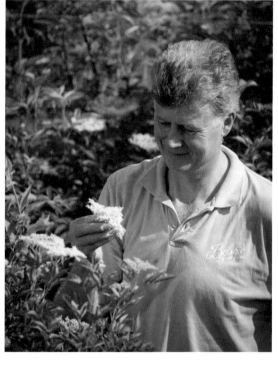

Jan Berry is a writer, herbalist, soap maker, and owner of the website *The Nerdy Farm Wife*. She's also the author of *Simple & Natural Soapmaking* and the *Big Book of Homemade Products*. She lives in the Blue Ridge Mountains of Virginia with her family where she enjoys collecting weeds and finding fun things to make with them. She's also an avid reader and enjoys nothing more than a good book and a cozy fire, with a purring kitty or snoring dog nearby.

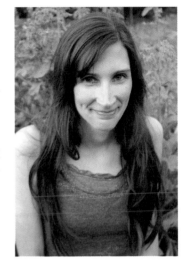

Bertrand Bouflet returned to his passion for gastronomy after twenty-eight years as a professional photographer, rediscovering the pleasure of making food and jams. Elderberry jelly (a recipe from his mother, Françoise) was at his table all year round. One evening his long-time friend Pierre-Louis suggested he make elderberry his business. It was a revelation. He decided to make elderberry a companion, an accomplice, and a partner for the next few years. He realized that no one in his region had really tested or developed elderberry to its potential, and the adventure really began. La Maison du Sureau now sells a line of quality jams, drinks, confections, and condiments following traditional recipes.

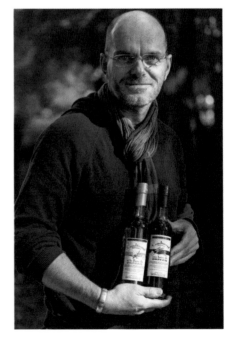

Chris Dalziel (pronounced Dee-EL) is a writer, researcher, and herbalist who helps natural moms create a homegrown lifestyle so they can shift away from the corporate health paradigm and create natural health and wellness within their family. Chris is the author of three books: *The Beeswax Workshop: How to Make Your Own Natural Candles, Cosmetics, Cleaners, Soaps, Healing Balms, and More,* 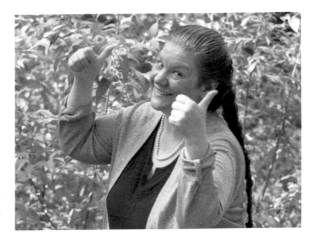 as well as *Homegrown Healing: From Seed to Apothecary,* and *The Beginner's Book of Essential Oils.* She is the founder of the JoybileeFarm.com blog and the founder and CEO of the membership site The DIY Herbal Fellowship.

Ben Doherty and **Erin Johnson** own Open Hands Farm, a certified organic seventeen-acre vegetable farm in Northfield, Minnesota. They are committed to feeding their community the freshest, most nutritious produce, grown in the most sustainable ways possible. Growing over 270 varieties of vegetables, fruits, flowers, and herbs, they also collaborate with two neighboring farms to make herbal products through Prairie Fire Herbal.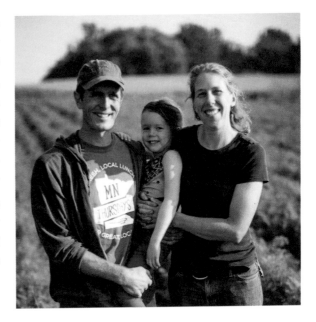

Chrystal Johnson is the author of the popular lifestyle blog, *Happy Mothering*, where she has been sharing her family's natural living journey since 2009. She lives in the mountains of Big Bear Lake, California, with her husband Brian and their two daughters, Zoë and Kaylee. Chrystal loves creating unique content for women on topics like DIY beauty, natural remedies, gluten-free recipes, homemaking, family travel, self-improvement, and more. When Chrystal isn't busy writing and creating inspiring content for her readers, you'll find her spending time with her family on the trails or by the lake. She finds her inspiration in nature and spends as much time outdoors as possible.

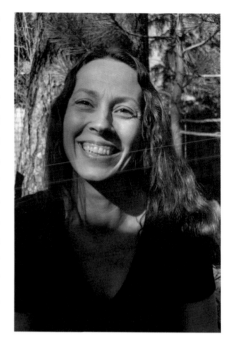

The Herbal Academy's mission is to teach the art and science of herbalism, honoring our intrinsic connection to nature. Dedicated to teaching and promoting a lifestyle of wellness and vitality through the use of herbs, sound nutrition, and optimal health practices, the Herbal Academy offers high-quality, affordable herbal studies programs to empower students and celebrate the community-centered spirit of herbalism by collaborating with a wide diversity of herbalists to present many herbal traditions and points of view. The Herbal Academy is committed to providing a path for herbal studies for those interested in personal development or a career in herbal medicine and to supporting their students all along their way.

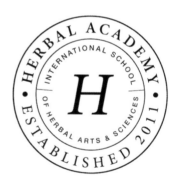

Carol Little, RH, is a traditional herbalist in Toronto, Canada, where she has a private practice working primarily with women. She has a unique system for helping her clients integrate holistic healing choices into their lives while helping them to move towards optimum health. Carol writes an herb-infused blog filled with seasonal tidbits, helpful hints, and ways to embrace herbs and healing foods, studiobotanica.com. She offers a seasonal newsletter with additional recipes and ideas for living an herbalicious life! Carol has written two popular ebooks: *Cold + Flu Season: Are YOU Ready?* and *Herbal Teas for Winter Health.* She is a past board member and current professional member of the Ontario Herbalists Association. She writes a chapter each year in the *Herb of the Year* book for the International Herb Association and is a contributing author for the *Home Herbalist* magazine. Follow her on social media @studiobotanica.

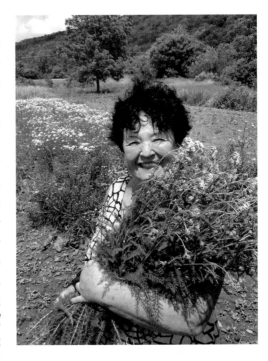

Anna Merhalski is a homesteading mama, garlic-worshipping foodie, and health research junkie. She lives on a small Maine homestead, surrounded by sheep, ducks, chickens, an enormous garden, and two happy, country-livin' kids. She blogs about it all over at SaltinmyCoffee.com

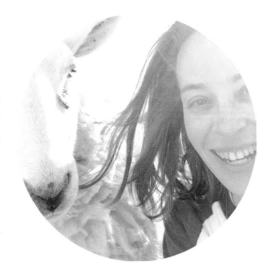

Vladka Merva discovered her passion for herbs, natural remedies, and beauty products when she moved to the alpine region in Switzerland. Long walks in the mountains surrounded by beautiful nature helped her uncover her real passion. She went back to her pharmaceutical science books and started to experiment and create herbal recipes, remedies, and beauty products. Later she launched *Simply Beyond Herbs*, a website that quickly won the hearts of many readers.

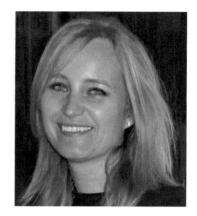

Ariana Mullins is an American writer, cook, explorer, and experimenter, and shares her family's stories of challenge and adventure as expats in Europe (currently in Southern Spain), as well as inspiration for living a simple and meaningful life. She has a passion for restoring lost kitchen arts and loves to share her experiences in foraging, butchery, home brewing, and anything new she can get her hands on through her website, *And Here We Are*, as well as her cookbook, *And Here We Are At the Table*.

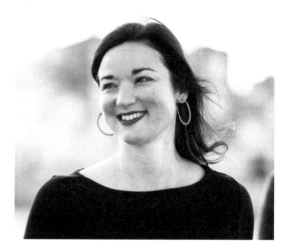

Laurie Neverman is the creator of *Common Sense Home*, one of the most popular self-reliance sites on the Internet. From professional caterer to operator of the world's largest flat plate solar water heating system, her skills cover a wide range of experience. She was a featured speaker at the Naval War College Strategic Studies Group, and has written for publications such as *Permaculture North America* and *Countryside* magazine. Her gardening adventures include permaculture, companion planting, vertical gardening, greenhouse cultivation, herbalism, and wildcrafting.

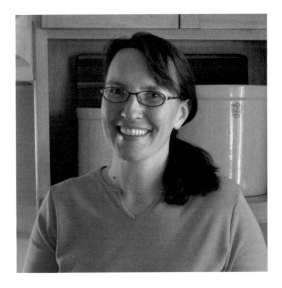

Norm's Farms is the nation's first vertically integrated three-family business focused entirely on the American elderberry. They take the elderberries grown sustainably on their family farms and turn them into delicious jams, flower syrups, and nutritional supplements using only natural, simple, and pure ingredients. You can find their products online at normsfarms. com, Amazon, and at select health food and grocery stores in more than thirty states. Visit their "Where to Buy" page to find the store nearest you!

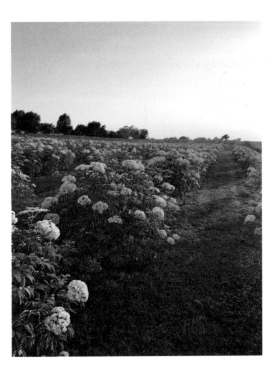

Loon Liquor Company was cofounded in 2013 by Simeon Rossi with Mark Schiller. The company aims to craft the most delicious spirits from organic, local suppliers while quantifiably improving social and environmental sustainability, and throwing in some humor from time to time. The name Loon Liquor represents not only their love of Minnesota

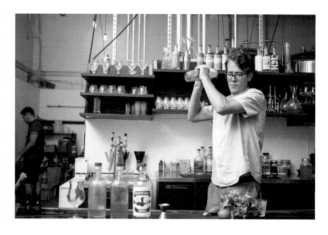

and its state bird, but also their commitment to preserving its natural habitat and the habitats of all endangered wildlife. Loon Liquor Company produces a wide assortment of spirits, including whiskey, vodka, gin, rum, and a line-up of flavorful liqueurs.

Hank Shaw, a lifelong forager, is the author of four award-winning cookbooks, most recently *Pheasant, Quail, Cottontail*, which won the IACP Award for best self-published book in 2019. He also runs the James Beard Award-winning website *Hunter Angler Gardener Cook* (huntgathercook.com). Shaw has been featured on numerous television shows, including Travel Channel's *Bizarre Foods* and CNN's *Somebody's Gotta Do It* with Mike Rowe. His work has appeared in *Food & Wine*, *Organic Gardening*, *Field & Stream*, *Garden & Gun*, and *The Art of Eating*. He hunts, fishes, and forages near Sacramento, California. Find him on social media @huntgathercook.

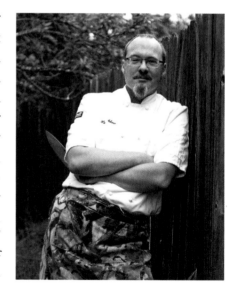

Heidi Skoog is the proprietor of Serious Jam. After nearly two decades as an award-winning florist, she swapped blooms for an apron to pursue her passion for food. A self-taught jam-maker, Heidi combines traditional methods and a flair for experimenting with flavor combinations and unusual ingredients. The result is a well-balanced, vibrant preserve that has a lot of love and story in every jar. Unexpected flavor combinations, such as Blueberry Bourbon Sage, Chai Spiced Pear Butter, and Meyer Lemon Earl Grey Marmalade have put Serious Jam on the culinary map. In addition to being serious about jam, Heidi is equally committed to teaching others to preserve the harvest, 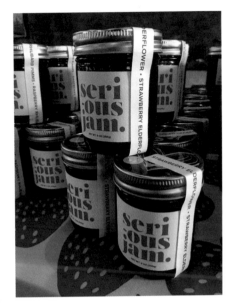 using food and herbs to heal, and testing her theories of kitchen-witchery on her super swell husband Kern and eager friends. Heidi and Kern can often be found slinging jam at farmer's markets together.

RECOMMENDED RESOURCES & FURTHER READING

Herbalism books:
Alchemy of Herbs by Rosalee de la Forêt
Backyard Herbal Apothecary by Devon Young
Body Into Balance by Maria Groves
The Earthwise Herbal by Matthew Wood
The Green Pharmacy by James Duke
The Herbal Apothecary by JJ Pursell
The Herbal Kitchen by Kami McBride
Making Plant Medicine by Richo Cech
Medicinal Herbs: A Beginner's Guide and *Herbs for Vital Health* by Rosemary Gladstar
The Modern Herbal Dispensatory, by Thomas Easley

Foraging Guides:
Identifying & Harvesting Edible and Medicinal Plants by Steve Brill
Nature's Garden by Samuel Thayer

Herbal Websites
Healing Harvest Homestead, healingharvesthomestead.com
The Herbal Academy, theherbalacademy.com
Herbs with Rosalee, herbalremediesadvice.org
Learning Herbs, learningherbs.com
Maud Grieves, *A Modern Herbal,* botanical.com/botanical/mgmh/mgmh.html
Nitty Gritty Life, nittygrittylife.com

Foraging Websites
Eat the Weeds, eattheweeds.com
Edible Wild Food, ediblewildfood.com
Grow Forage Cook Ferment, growforagecookferment.com
Practical Self Reliance, practicalselfreliance.com
"Wildman" Steve Brill, wildmanstevebrill.com

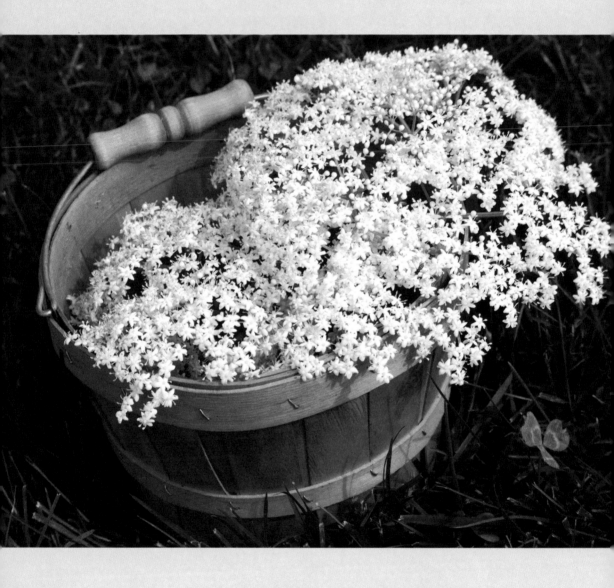

ACKNOWLEDGMENTS

I want to thank all the people who helped make this book happen, beginning with Leah Zarra, my editor at Skyhorse, who invited me to submit a proposal.

A HUGE thank you to Erin Johnson and Ben Doherty of Open Hands Farm for sharing not only their favorite recipes but the bountiful elderflowers and berries growing on their farm. Thanks also to the numerous elderberry growers and researchers—Andrew Thomas, Patrick Byers, Terry Durham, Brent Madding, Chris Patton, Aaron Wills, Devon Bennett, and Ann Lenhardt—who shared their elderberry wisdom with me.

Rosalee de la Forêt and Lise Wolff were a tremendous help talking to me about how they use elderberries in their practices. Researchers Peter Valtchev, Daniel Lubahn, and Alice Jones patiently explained to me the ins and outs of their investigations.

Gratitude to Sim Rossi of Loon Liquor for talking to me at length about elderflowers and to Heidi Skoog for sharing her jam-making. And to all the innovative bloggers and food-experimenters who contributed recipes to this book.

A big thanks to my family for thinking some of my forays into foraging and herbal medicine were not simply odd, but occasionally kind of cool. (And even agreeing to try a few of them!) Thanks especially to my mother, Carole Shmurak, for reading drafts and consulting on chemistry, and to Annette Jarman for loaning me countless props for my photographs. I am also greatly indebted to my husband, Baird, who offered feedback on drafts, talked over ideas, advised on numerous issues, *and* looked after the kids while I went off foraging, researching, and writing. And never complained about the many messes I made in the kitchen!

And most of all, to the ever-growing herbal community, who shares centuries-old herbal wisdom in decidedly modern ways. I am always learning from them.

CONVERSION CHARTS

METRIC AND IMPERIAL CONVERSIONS
(These conversions are rounded for convenience)

Ingredient	Cups/Tablespoons/Teaspoons	Ounces	Grams/Milliliters
Butter	1 cup/ 16 tablespoons/ 2 sticks	8 ounces	230 grams
Cheese, shredded	1 cup	4 ounces	110 grams
Cream cheese	1 tablespoon	0.5 ounce	14.5 grams
Cornstarch	1 tablespoon	0.3 ounce	8 grams
Flour, all-purpose	1 cup/1 tablespoon	4.5 ounces/0.3 ounce	125 grams/8 grams
Flour, whole wheat	1 cup	4 ounces	120 grams
Fruit, dried	1 cup	4 ounces	120 grams
Fruits or veggies, chopped	1 cup	5 to 7 ounces	145 to 200 grams
Fruits or veggies, pureed	1 cup	8.5 ounces	245 grams
Honey, maple syrup, or corn syrup	1 tablespoon	0.75 ounce	20 grams
Liquids: cream, milk, water, or juice	1 cup	8 fluid ounces	240 milliliters
Oats	1 cup	5.5 ounces	150 grams
Salt	1 teaspoon	0.2 ounce	6 grams
Spices: cinnamon, cloves, ginger, or nutmeg (ground)	1 teaspoon	0.2 ounce	5 milliliters
Sugar, brown, firmly packed	1 cup	7 ounces	200 grams
Sugar, white	1 cup/1 tablespoon	7 ounces/0.5 ounce	200 grams/12.5 grams
Vanilla extract	1 teaspoon	0.2 ounce	4 grams

OVEN TEMPERATURES

Fahrenheit	Celsius	Gas Mark
225°	110°	¼
250°	120°	½
275°	140°	1
300°	150°	2
325°	160°	3
350°	180°	4
375°	190°	5
400°	200°	6
425°	220°	7
450°	230°	8

INDEX